THRIVING MOVING FORWARD

THRIVING MOVING FORWARD

A GUIDE TO HEALTHY AGING

Debbye Omlie and Blake Anderson

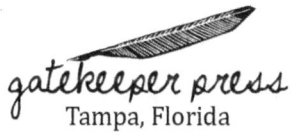
Tampa, Florida

The views and opinions expressed in this book are solely those of the author and do not reflect the views or opinions of Gatekeeper Press. Gatekeeper Press is not to be held responsible for and expressly disclaims responsibility of the content herein.

THRIVING MOVING FORWARD:
A Guide to Healthy Aging

Published by Gatekeeper Press
7853 Gunn Hwy, Suite 209
Tampa, FL 33626
www.GatekeeperPress.com

Copyright © 2024 by Debbye Omlie and Blake Anderson

All rights reserved. Neither this book, nor any parts within it may be sold or reproduced in any form or by any electronic or mechanical means, including information storage and retrieval systems, without permission in writing from the author. The only exception is by a reviewer, who may quote short excerpts in a review.

The cover design, interior formatting, typesetting, and editorial work for this book are entirely the product of the author. Gatekeeper Press did not participate in and is not responsible for any aspect of these elements.

Library of Congress Control Number: 2024932965

ISBN (paperback): 9781662945243
eISBN: 9781662945250

Table of Contents

FOREWORD BY T. COLIN CAMPBELL, PHD	1
INTRODUCTION BY DEBBYE OMLIE	3
Need to Recalibrate Expectations Around Aging	3
Health Is Real Wealth	3
My Story	4
Self-Responsibility for My Health & Wellness	6
If Not Now, When?	7
Why Should You Read the Book?	8
INTRODUCTION BY BLAKE ANDERSON	11
My Health	11
My Tragedy	13
My New Life	15
Back to the Book	16
1. THE ART OF START	19
Where Do You Want to Go?	19
Where Are You Starting From?	20
What Is Your Path?	20
What Do You Need to Start Your Journey?	21
What Will You Need to Support You on the Way?	21
2. BUILDING A HEALTH-CARE TEAM	23
Primary Care Provider (PCP)	23
How Can You Find a PCP?	24
The Rest of Your Health-Care Team	25
Benefits of Wellness Coaching	26
Track Your Health and Take Control	28

3. YOUR EMOTIONAL AND MENTAL LIFE 31
    Intuitive Wisdom 32
    Designing a Thriving Life 33
    Small Habits Make Big Changes 33
    Growth Mindset 34
    Ways to Manage Stress 35
    Attitude of Gratitude 36
    The Power of Resilience 37
    Restorative Sleep 37
    Keep Building Your Brain & Increase Your Cognitive Reserve
    with Lifelong Learning 39
    Do You Play? 40
    Importance of Connections and Engagement 42
    What Can We Do When Our Network Isn't Supportive? ... 42
    Feeling Stuck? 43

4. SO WHY DO YOU WANT TO LIVE LONGER? 47
    Rekindling an Old Passion 48
    Same Job, Different Attitudes 49
    Help Fix the Planet 50
    Quality of Life 50

5. YOUR NUTRITIONAL LIFE 53
    Four Dietary Patterns Associated with Reducing Chronic
    Disease Today 54
    What Is a Whole Food, Plant-Based (WFPB) Diet? 54
    Can Food Prevent Alzheimer's Disease? 56
    WFPB Diet Put to the Test. The Power of Food Over COVID-19 ... 56
    Can a WFPB Diet Reverse Cancer? 57
    How to Learn to Cook WFPB Meals 57

6. HOW AND WHY OTHERS STARTED ON THE WFPB PATH 59
    Meet Rod Horn 59
    Meet Chris Kalinich 61
    Meet Amanda Strombom 64
    Meet Gigi Carter 67

7.	YOUR PHYSICAL LIFE	71
	Gotta Move More & Sit Less	72
	Exercise Lengthens Telomeres and Your Life	73
	What Constitutes Aerobic Exercise?	74
	Strength Training Is Important as We Age	74
	How Much and How Long?	75
	What is the Difference Between Moderate and Vigorous Aerobic Activity?	75
	The Benefits of Simple Walking	76
	Ready to Run a Marathon?	77
	Carter Incorporates Exercise into Her Healthy Lifestyle	78
8.	ENVIRONMENT MATTERS	81
	Do You Live in a Soul-Nourishing Space?	81
	Setting Your Environment Up for Success	82
	Minimize Exposure to Toxins	83
	Ways to Avoid Environmental Chemicals in Your Food	85
	Additional Protection Against Environmental Chemicals	85
	Toxic Ingredients in Skin Care Products	86
	Your Virtual World	87
9.	BEAUTY REDEFINED	91
	A Different Way to Think About Beauty	91
10.	CONCLUSION	95
	Time to Create Your Customized Plan	95
	Your Customized Plan	96
	Go Back and Review the Chapters	97
RESOURCES		99
ENDNOTES		105
ACKNOWLEDGEMENTS		115
ABOUT DEBBYE		117
ABOUT BLAKE		119

FOREWORD BY
T. Colin Campbell, PhD

Debbye Omlie says it right and has chosen a select audience with whom she has the experience to share her story and how it might be used. It's about the kind of food we choose to eat, suitable for virtually any lifestyle we may find within our surroundings.

I am convinced of the veracity of her story. As a professional scientist for more than six decades, I became profoundly fascinated with this idea because of its underlying science, because of my struggle to change my own biases and habits acquired during my youth, and because of the proactive efforts made by professionals and authorities for well over a century to deny this story to the larger audience for self-serving purposes. Mainly, the diet that Debbye espouses works for people of all ages, ultimately preventing and even reversing ailments that increasingly appear as we age.

I suggest that this book has the capacity to affect health as much or more than any other course of action we might wish to take. It also has meaning for issues well beyond our personal lives. I speak of its ability to decrease health care costs and to help us save our environment, indeed, our planet. These are huge stories that must be told.

T. Colin Campbell, PhD
Jacob Gould Schurman Professor
Emeritus of Nutritional Biochemistry
Cornell University
Co-author of *The China Study*, the New York Times best-seller, *Whole*, and *The Future of Nutrition*

WHY AM I WRITING THIS BOOK?
Introduction By Debbye Omlie

Need to Recalibrate Expectations Around Aging

We need a new conversation around aging that includes the word "thriving." In this period of history, we are in an aging revolution. We are living longer. Over seventy million baby boomers are living out this fact. It's time to reimagine healthy aging as a state of thriving instead of declining. We can't stop aging, but we can control *how* we age. Otherwise, we are leaving a lot of our lives in the hands of fate. So, it's time to take charge of our health and life!

Healthy aging is the result of a healthy lifestyle, plain and simple.

Most people agree that "healthy" is important. But how exactly does "healthy" happen? And what does "healthy" really involve? I propose most people don't know what healthy means in today's world, let alone how to control their health. I didn't.

Health Is Real Wealth

It is hard to have a great life without good health. Yet most people only think about their health after they receive a difficult diagnosis. Other than that, many people pretty much ignore their health. "It is unfortunate that so few appreciate from what small causes diseases come,"[1] said Dr. Charles Mayo, co-founder of the Mayo Clinic. But why is this information being ignored?

Many people believe that they are doomed to decline based on the genes they inherited. However, the plethora of research shows clearly that your genes only constitute up to a 20 percent risk of inherited disease(s).

How we decline is up to us. We control more than we think.

My Story

I am not a celebrity or even a medical professional, just a woman who found a way to thrive more than decline in her sixties. I drew a line in the sand and said, "No more!" I am going to do this my way. I will figure it out! Losing my family to cancer and Alzheimer's disease (lifestyle-related chronic diseases that could have been avoided), I knew there had to be a better way to age. So, my search began, and aha moments came marching in.

Health and wellness aren't new to me. Over thirty years ago, I created a worksite wellness program for a Honeywell division, heralded by the American Heart Association as a model in New Mexico, and that project began my interest in good health practices. As a result, I have worked in numerous health organizations promoting healthy living principles and practices. Unfortunately, through the years, I have been on and (mostly) off the path. And it would take a series of difficult life events for me to start making changes.

Five years into my search, my primary care provider (PCP) wanted to put me on statins because of a borderline high cholesterol issue. It was a barely borderline issue. And one I had had for years. I was an unhealthy ethical vegetarian. While I didn't eat meat, I did eat processed foods, sugar, oil, and dairy. When I declined his offer for statins, he suggested that I read *Food Rules* by Michael Pollan. I knew I didn't need to be convinced of the power of plants.

Instead, I needed to understand what I was doing wrong (which he couldn't tell me). He also suggested I see a dietician. I declined that offer, as I suspected animal products would be encouraged.

At the time, I was working full time at a very demanding job with a long commute and helping to care for my dad, who was suffering from Alzheimer's disease. To say I was stressed out would be an understatement.

But change is the only constant in our lives. I needed to make peace with that fact and see health and aging differently.

In an aha moment during this period, I connected to the thought that the definition of beauty also needs to change as we age. It was time to accept aging on my terms! This quote by Maya Angelou kept coming to me: "We delight in the beauty of the butterfly, but rarely admit the changes it has gone through to achieve that beauty." Finally, I understood that I needed to also see beauty not through the popular cultural definition—youth as beauty—but through the changes. Not a popular concept in today's world. More about this in Chapter 9, Beauty Redefined.

I also learned that self-care isn't selfish. And it wasn't about pedicures and massages, although those were nice indulgences. For me, self-care needed to be much deeper and more robust than that. After thinking about it, I made a list of the changes that were needed to take care of me as I aged.

With all that I was going through and had been through, I realized that I had developed wisdom as I aged. And with that wisdom, self-care needed to encompass:

- Taking responsibility for my health and wellness
- Analyzing my emotional/mental life, nutritional life, and physical life annually and making the necessary changes to be healthy
- Evaluating the environment that I live in and making the necessary changes to create a soul-nourishing one centered around wellness
- Building a healthcare team that I can communicate with, feel heard by, and trust

- Saying no to the things that deplete me (people, jobs, activities, and situations) and yes to the ones that nourish me

- Understanding that beauty is an inside job

It was time to embrace the need to make changes.

Self-Responsibility for My Health & Wellness

Soon after my conversation with my PCP, I watched the *Forks Over Knives* documentary. It convinced me that I, not the medical establishment, was responsible for my health! This was another aha moment. And I needed to take charge! My health was too valuable to give the responsibility over to someone else, like my PCP, and take the recommended prescription drugs. Instead, I needed to work with my PCP as a partner, not follow his instructions blindly. Until I understood this point, I didn't get it. I wouldn't make the necessary changes to be healthy because it takes work, sacrifice, and dedication.

As Albert Einstein said, "The world as we have created it is a process of our thinking. It cannot be changed without changing our thinking." This thought kept running through my head. It was time for me to rethink the entire aging process.

The next profound thing to happen was hearing two neurologists, Ayesha and Dean Sherzai, MDs, from Loma Linda, California (the only Blue Zone in the US), discuss how to prevent and reverse Alzheimer's disease. The presentation was based on the research they were involved in. Both doctors serve as co-directors of the Alzheimer's Prevention Program at Loma Linda University Medical Center. Blue Zones are areas where people don't eat like typical Americans and live longer and healthier because of it.

Finally, I was starting to hear *ways to prevent* that dreaded disease. Another aha moment. Hearing them was another game changer for me. I now knew that I was on the right path.

As a result of the changes that I have made, I lowered my cholesterol to a healthy range within six months. My biometric numbers steadily improved, so much so that one of my doctors commented he wished he had them. I cleared up migraines and digestive issues that had harassed me for years. A problem that I have had in one of my eyes significantly improved, and my ophthalmologist attributed it to "what I was eating." Also, I lost over thirty pounds and have kept it off to this day. As a result, I continue to feel the best I have ever felt in my life, with enormous energy. And I am healthier and fitter in my sixties than I was in my forties.

If Not Now, When?

It is time to take responsibility and control of your health and not just complacently assume your genes dictate your fate and that you are therefore doomed to suffer from chronic disease(s) and the side effects from the pills used to manage them. Fortunately, 80 percent of chronic diseases are lifestyle-related and not a normal part of aging. That means you can prevent or reverse them in many cases.[2]

We live in one of the wealthiest countries in the world with a population of some of the unhealthiest.[3] A CDC report states that 78 percent of Americans (women and men) aged fifty-five years and over suffer from at least one chronic disease.[4] And 47 percent (almost half) have been diagnosed with two or more.[5] Today, when it comes to chronic diseases, heart disease is the number one killer and kills more women than men.[6] Cancer is the second. And COVID-19 is now the third leading cause of death in the US. According to a CDC report, those affected by COVID-19 and "living with a chronic disease were six times more likely to be hospitalized and twelve times more likely to die" from January to the end of May 2020.[7]

Unfortunately, suffering from a chronic disease and the side effects of the drugs used to manage it is now the norm. "We medicate ourselves with toxic concoctions, a small number of which treat the disease, while the rest treat the harmful effects of the primary drugs,"[8] states T. Colin Campbell, PhD.

Chronic diseases are broadly defined as issues lasting one year or more and requiring ongoing attention and/or limiting activities of daily living or both. Chronic diseases such as heart disease, cancer, and diabetes are the leading causes of death and disability in the United States, according to the CDC. Others include chronic lung disease, stroke, Alzheimer's disease, and chronic kidney disease.

To be clear, I am not saying that you need to stop taking your pills and medications. I am saying you should take control of your health. And I am suggesting that you approach this book with a curiosity about the possibility of reversing or preventing chronic disease. Also, I am not saying don't use medicine or medical care. When you need it, use it, especially in emergency situations. Please know that you can take charge of your health and start making changes daily that can lead to better results long-term. And always discuss options with your PCP.

Why Should You Read the Book?

This book describes my journey, what I discovered, and, more importantly, put into practice. And it has taken me years. This is not some fad found on the internet. Instead, I share scientific, evidence-based information (with citations) that I have used. While there are no guarantees, there is much data to suggest that we have a better chance of living longer and thriving by trying many of the suggestions. I found there are many aspects that need to be considered besides diet and exercise. Instead, it is an entire lifestyle. The need to prevent chronic diseases and the ways to prevent them are woven throughout this book.

I share areas to focus on in partnership with your PCP. With this knowledge, you don't have to be a victim of the aging process or the Standard American Diet/Western diet (fried foods, sugar, oils, dairy, processed foods, processed meats, animal and fowl meat, and refined grains). Instead, you hold the power to age, thriving one day at a time.

You have control over the small choices you make every day:

- What you eat and drink
- Your thoughts and how you react to stress
- The amount of quality sleep you get
- How and when you exercise
- Your friends and support group
- Your environment
- Living out your purpose

And all the above affect your immune system. A healthy immune system is important to your overall health and wellness, especially with the threat of pandemics and other viruses.

What you are reading is a beginner's manual for anyone who wants to age gracefully. It is the book I was trying to find and couldn't years ago. It contains the information you need to create a customized health plan for yourself. I call it a manual because I want you to think of it as a handbook or set of instructions on aging gracefully with an emphasis on your health.

Because this book serves as an introduction to how to be healthy from a 30,000-foot level, it is beyond the scope of this book to dive deeply into the topics. Instead, I hope to stir your curiosity by sharing different areas that affect health and aging well. You can then decide if you need to deep dive into more information. A full list of resources is provided at the book's end for further exploration. I present the information in the most succinct, logical way to understand it.

This book initially started out for women. However, after I sent it out for comments, my mind quickly changed. Men needed (and were interested) in hearing the message, 100 percent of the readers said. As a result, I invited Blake to co-author not only for his male perspective but also for his training and experience as a Mayo Clinic-trained wellness coach. And the book is much more informative with his addition.

So, while it is tempting to blame genetics, the medical establishment, or anything else, it is best to be honest. What is holding you back from living the healthiest and best life you can have?

WHY AM I CO-WRITING THIS BOOK?
Introduction by Blake Anderson

My Health

My own health journey began when I was about forty. As an adolescent and young adult, I had always been tall and thin. Fast-forward to forty, and I recall being faced with the prospect of, for the first time in my life, buying jeans where the waist size exceeded the length. I don't know why, but for some reason I considered this to be a "point of no return." That, if I crossed that line, it would then become acceptable, and I would never drop that weight. Prior to that time, I'd never watched my weight. I had seemingly been able to eat whatever I wanted with no repercussions. I'm not sure when that changed, but it clearly snuck up on me.

I was playing basketball once a week, so I considered myself somewhat active. However, I had chronic knee pain, bringing a cooler of ice packs with me to wear on my knees during the drive home from the gym. In addition, of course, to the ice pack on my lower back. It would take me almost a week to recover before doing it all over again. At the time, I thought this was a natural outcome of aging. I was forty after all. I can't feel young and spry forever.

It was the weight that was bothering me, though, so I decided to do something about it. I didn't want to go on a diet because I knew that diets simply don't work. So, I skipped that step and moved directly to figuring out some permanent lifestyle changes that I would need to make. I started with a food log, listing everything that I consumed, food and drink, along with the calorie content. Wow, was that ever an eye opener! I'm embarrassed to say, looking back on it, that I was consuming around four to six cans of full-calorie Coke every day. At 140 calories each, that was adding 560 to 840 calories per day. That's the equivalent of adding an extra full meal on top of what I was already eating. No wonder my weight had ballooned! And just like that, the first habit I needed to change was staring me right in the face.

In addition to dropping full-calorie sodas, I decided that I would not consume any calories from beverages at all (goodbye, morning orange juice) because I felt that the nutritional density of anything I could drink was not worth the calorie content. Today, my staple drink is zero-calorie seltzer water. I drink a cup of black coffee every morning. I will occasionally drink a diet soda, but my palate now finds that too sweet to drink consistently.

I made some other relatively minor changes to the way I ate that had significant impacts on my overall calorie consumption. I eliminated high-calorie "sides" when going out to eat. I might get a hamburger, but I won't get fries. I will eat a sandwich, but I won't add chips. I opt for steamed vegetables over mashed potatoes. This step alone can cut calories in a meal by 20–50 percent without sacrificing the things that satisfy my hunger and my tastes. I reduced my portion sizes, ordering single-patty hamburgers and half-sandwiches. I opted for hearty salads, like a salmon Caesar, over heavier entrees. I also switched higher-calorie sauces and condiments for lower-calorie options. Mustard over mayonnaise, marinara over cream sauce, vinaigrette over ranch. For me, these did not significantly change my enjoyment of these foods but did significantly change the number of calories I was consuming.

In addition to this, I increased my activity level. I walked nearly every day for at least thirty to sixty minutes. I added weight training to my regimen. As my activity level and strength increased, my weight dropped. I was able to add another day of basketball to my week, and my recovery time dropped. I was able to add another day or two of basketball without the need to ice my joints or take anti-inflammatory medications.

After about two years, I had dropped over fifty pounds, and I have kept it off to this day, over ten years later. Again, not because I went on some temporary diet but because I'd made lifestyle changes that would stand the test of time. Now I'm able to maintain my weight without thinking about it because my eating habits and my activity level support the weight that I'm at with literally no effort on my part.

In writing this book with Debbye, I see the value of a whole-food, plant-based (WFPB) diet. The health benefits of adopting such a diet are quite clear to me. I'm moving in that direction, but I'm not personally convinced that I'll ever make it there. Why do I say this? Because you don't have to make a wholesale change to make a difference in your life. You can make small, subtle changes that start to move you in the direction that you want to go. Once you establish a new set of habits that are healthier for you, you can consider what additional small changes you would like to make. But that second set of changes is being made from a healthier baseline, so these changes compound. You can repeat this pattern until you ultimately get to where you want to be. If you can make a wholesale switch to WFPB, that's great! If not, what if you doubled your fruits and vegetables and cut your meat in half? You're still better off.

My Tragedy

In the midst of my battle with weight (hindsight suggesting the following was probably a non-negligible contributor to that), I was dealing with a crushing blow in my personal life. My wife of almost ten years, Laura, was diagnosed with brain cancer.

In late 2001, Laura was plagued by headaches that were so bad she couldn't get out of bed for days. She could not keep food or liquid down, and merely changing positions in bed would cause her to vomit. With a family history of migraine headaches, the doctor was quick to diagnose. While medications didn't work right away, the headaches would eventually subside. And then return.

In late December of that year, she fainted in the shower. This was so concerning that we decided to push for her to get an MRI. It was a Thursday afternoon, and the MRI procedure itself went well. We were told the results would be forthcoming. When we returned home from dinner later that evening, we were greeted by an ominous message from her doctor on our answering machine: "I need to see you and Blake in my office tomorrow at 5:00 p.m."

I spent the following night awake, tossing and turning. I spent the next day scouring the internet, looking for anything that suggested that this could be anything other than something really, really bad. When we arrived at the doctor's office, the doctor told Laura, "We got the results back from your MRI, and it shows that you have a tumor in your brain. And it is big."

Meetings with an oncologist, radiologist, neurosurgeon, and more tests followed, and within a week of the MRI, she was on an operating table with doctors working to remove as much of the tumor as they could. They ended up removing about half of what they told us was an anaplastic astrocytoma from her right frontal lobe. The other half would have to be treated through a regimen of chemotherapy and radiation, as it was too dangerous to remove.

Following a couple rounds of the standard treatment, the tumor showed signs of progression. The doctors suggested that we continue down that path. Looking back, I realize that they weren't aiming to "cure" her but simply trying to buy her more time. Unsatisfied with this, in my naivete, I did some research and ended up enrolling her in a clinical trial at Duke University. Living on the West Coast meant transcontinental flights every eight weeks for a year, but it was worth the time and effort.

Laura's body struggled to tolerate the trial medications, so they transitioned her to another therapy, which was also challenging for her. Ultimately, in August of 2003, the doctors recommended that we stop treatment. Interestingly, by then, MRI scans were showing no progression of the cancer, so there was a sliver of a chance that she was out of the woods.

By this time, Laura had lost her job but was very interested in going back to work. We agreed that she could take on some light housework to start getting into the habit of being productive again. This revealed that there were other factors at play. She could never quite muster up the motivation to be productive. We worked with an occupational therapist and made no progress. She ended up having a neuropsychological evaluation, which indicated that she did have some impairment in the region of her brain that controls motivation and judgment.

Due largely to the lasting effects of the radiation treatment, this impairment progressed over the years, and I watched her abilities and her love for me slowly disappear one by one. In 2017, I finally made the excruciatingly difficult decision to move her into an assisted living facility where she could get the 24/7 care that she needed. While she is no longer able to walk or dress herself or care for herself in any way and her short-term memory is severely impaired, she is largely coherent and enjoys when I visit her a couple of times a week.

My New Life

It was 2008 when Laura first told me that she didn't love me anymore. I tried to regain her love but didn't realize until much later that it never had anything to do with me. This was tied directly to what was going on with her brain. I slowly began to realize that I was no longer her spouse, no longer her partner or friend. Now I was simply her caregiver. This was a shock to my system, as my whole identity was tied up in being a committed husband.

Somewhere along the line, I devised a ridiculous plan, a plan so outlandish that it seemed extremely unlikely to work. And yet a voice in my head kept telling me it was possible. What if I could find another partner? Someone who could accept where I was in my life. Someone who could see me as loyal and generous and kind and be someone willing and able to receive all the love I felt I had to give. So, I dove headfirst into the turbulent waters of online dating.

I met Brandi on April 15, 2018. We had coffee and went for a short, unseasonably cold walk under overcast skies around Green Lake that Sunday afternoon. We played squash together the following Friday, and I grilled some steaks and vegetables at my house for her on Saturday. I'd like to say that we were inseparable ever since, but there was a minor snag. She wanted a child. After years of caring for a disabled adult, I wanted freedom.

What followed was a back and forth, on-and-off romance that made it clear that even though we had different visions of our future, we had to stay together. Brandi moved into my house in September 2019, with the issue of children tabled for the time being.

The pandemic hit, and we were quarantined together. I swear that experience fast-forwarded our relationship at least five years. It brought us closer together than anything else I imagine could have. A shift happened for me during that time, and I began to open my heart to the possibility of having children.

I'm happy to say that our IVF journey was successful! Now, at fifty-three years old, I am about to become a first-time father within one month of me writing these words, appropriately, on Father's Day.

Back to the Book

Throughout these peaks and valleys, I started to recognize that there were aspects of my life that were tightly interconnected. I observed that difficulties in one area inevitably bled over to other areas. Likewise, when everything was going well across the board, I felt at peace. I also realized that I couldn't control the things that happened to me, but I could control how I reacted. I was able to shed the paralyzing self-pity that could have left me wallowing in my own misery and envisioned a better life for myself. Working toward that vision, I set forth making minor but meaningful and permanent changes to my habits and routines, turning small successes in each area of my life into huge gains for my overall well-being that persisted over time.

This is Wellness. I have a passion for it because I can clearly see how all of the dimensions of wellness are interconnected and that something which impacts one dimension, for good or for bad, will permeate through the others. I've also come to realize that paying keen attention to these dimensions and taking a proactive approach to addressing challenges helps to achieve and maintain wellness over the long haul. What I love most is that, due to the interconnected nature of wellness, improvements in one dimension impact the others, like a rising tide lifting all boats, and the effort you put in has a compounding effect.

I started Honu Perspective, my Life and Wellness Coaching practice, in 2021 as the fusion of my life experiences and my desire to help others. I have a wellness coaching certification from the Mayo Clinic and life coaching certifications from Elite Coaching University that have allowed me to develop the skills necessary to help guide others through their own journey. I teach people how to envision a future they want for themselves, identify what they need to do to get started, and establish processes and habits that keep them moving forward, persisting through the ups and downs of life. People feel more in control of their lives and choices and enjoy more happiness and fulfillment. What's more, with the skills that they've gained and the success that they've experienced, they feel more confident and empowered to live life on their terms.

It was through this new career development that I met Debbye. She told me about this book that she was writing and thought that I could contribute, providing a male perspective. Debbye has a boundless energy that belies her age, and it is my sincere honor to contribute to this book where she reveals exactly how she has managed to achieve that. Thanks, Debbye!

CHAPTER 1

The Art of Start

This first chapter covers a lot of ground at a high level. You will be asked to consider some very broad questions and take an honest accounting of your current health situation. But don't get overwhelmed! The rest of this book is here to help you fill in the blanks. And remember, the path to good health is a journey not a destination.

So, using the journey metaphor, this book is designed to help you answer the following questions:

1. Where do you want to go?
2. Where are you starting from?
3. What is your path?
4. What do you need to start your journey?
5. What will you need to support you along the way?

Where Do You Want to Go?

The art of start is to begin at the end. While the path to good health is a journey and not a destination, we still need to have a destination in mind. This will help guide you on the choices you make on your journey as inevitable roadblocks present themselves. This will help you stay on the right path. Otherwise, you end up wandering aimlessly.

Presumably, you are reading this book because health matters to you and you either want to achieve or maintain "good health." So, what does "good health" mean to you? What are you trying to achieve?

If you're struggling to answer that question, here's an exercise to help you: close your eyes and transport yourself to a year in the future. Now, imagine you've accomplished everything you set out to accomplish over the last year. Feeling that full sense of pride and achievement, as if it has already happened, write down all of your accomplishments. Congratulations! You now have a destination in mind!

Where Are You Starting From?

Well, it's kind of a silly answer, but right where you are! Before you can get somewhere, you have to know where you are starting from. So, using your present state of health as a basis, begin where you are and document your:

- Known risk factors
- Any chronic diseases you have (or health issues)
- Current biometric readings (height, weight, body mass index (BMI), blood pressure, blood cholesterol, and blood sugar)

And always work with your PCP before starting any recommendations in this book.

What Is Your Path?

You need to map it out for yourself. Your journey to good health consists of behavior changes that you need to make. There are three important components to health that you control to begin with:

- Nutrition
- Activity Level
- Sleep

This book provides ideas for healthy behaviors that will have you headed in the right direction.

Mapping out your path is a critical step in the process because the changes you make need to both get you on the road in the right direction of your destination *and* keep you on the road. That is, they need to align with your definition of "good health," and they need to be sustainable changes that you can make a permanent part of your lifestyle. Any changes that require willpower are not likely to stick, and you run the very real risk of becoming discouraged and veering off the road. That's not to say that the changes won't require some discipline, but the objective is to use the short-term discipline to establish new habits that last a lifetime.

What Do You Need to Start Your Journey?

What specific changes did you commit to? What will you need to support those changes? A gym membership? Some new walking shoes and/or custom orthotics from a podiatrist? An air fryer? Anything you need to make the changes you committed to easier and more likely to stick is what you should be considering. This book also highlights the importance of starting with a health-care team.

What Will You Need to Support You on the Way?

Emotional and mental health are interconnected with your physical health. You can't have one without the other, especially when it comes to making lifestyle changes and keeping yourself on track. You will invariably encounter hurdles and roadblocks along the way. Healthy emotional and mental states will enable you to persevere in the face of these obstacles. This book also delves into the importance of a supportive environment.

IMPORTANT DISCLAIMER: Please be aware that this book's materials and content are for general information only and are not intended to be a substitute for professional medical advice, diagnosis, or treatment. Readers of this book should not rely on the information provided for their own health needs. All specific questions should be presented to your healthcare provider(s).

CHAPTER 2

Building a Health-Care Team

Primary Care Provider (PCP)

A PCP is essential to your well-being, and you might be surprised at how many people don't realize this. You may think to yourself, "I never get sick" or "I just use specialists when I need them." Or maybe even "I have one, but I don't like him/her." If you don't already have a PCP (even if you don't presently need one or don't like the one you have), now is the time to find one you like and feel comfortable with!

A PCP, also called a family doctor, can be such a valuable resource, especially when you find one that takes time to get to know you. It will establish a good foundation for providing excellent care over the rest of your life.

The PCP serves as the quarterback of your health-care team. Because a PCP is trained in all areas of medicine, a PCP is best qualified to help you navigate a successful and productive health-care journey. A good one will listen, make notes about your health history, and understand your nuances, beliefs, preferences, values, life stages, and current situations. As a result, your PCP can help you make really good decisions about your health.

As the quarterback, your PCP is also responsible for diagnosing and treating issues like headaches, back pain, and urinary infections. Your PCP also supervises chronic conditions like high blood pressure, diabetes, heart disease, obesity, anxiety, and depression. And your PCP advises you about routine screenings, shots, vaccinations, and decisions about lifestyle changes.[1]

Communication is key to a good relationship with your PCP.

The National Institute on Aging advises:

> Finding the main doctor (often called your primary care doctor) to whom you feel comfortable talking is the first step in good communication. How well you and your doctor talk to each other is one of the most important steps in getting good healthcare. The doctor gets to know you and what your health is normally like.
>
> Taking an active role in your health puts the responsibility for good communication on both you and your doctor. This means asking questions if the doctor's explanations or instructions are unclear, bringing up problems even if the doctor doesn't ask, and letting the doctor know you have concerns about a particular treatment or change in your daily life.[2]

It is time to find a new doctor if you don't have a PCP or are not comfortable with the one you currently see.

How Can You Find a PCP?

You can start with recommendations from family and friends to help you identify one. Or see if your insurance company has a list of PCPs in their network, advises familydoctor.org. Next, call the office to find out:

- Is the physician board-certified in family practice?
- Are they taking new patients?
- Do they take your insurance (if not determined before)?
- What are their office hours?
- Do they accept walk-ins after hours?
- Do they have on-call hours?
- What is the average time to get an appointment with a doctor?
- What hospital does the doctor use?
- How many doctors are in the practice?
- Do they perform labs and imaging in the office? If not, do they refer patients to a place that is in your insurance network?

Happy with the answers? Now you can make an appointment!

At the appointment, try to decide:

- Was the office easy to get to?
- Did the office staff seem friendly and likable?
- Was the check-in process smooth?
- Were you comfortable with the doctor?
- Did the doctor answer all of your questions?
- Was the doctor interested in getting to know you?
- Did the doctor explain things so you could understand?
- Was the office clean?
- Was the doctor patient with you?[3]

Also consider asking questions like:

- Do you have many older patients?
- How do you feel about involving my family in care decisions?
- Can I call or email you or your staff when I have questions? Do you charge for telephone or email time?
- What telehealth services do you offer?
- What are your thoughts about complementary or alternative treatments, such as . . .?[4]

Selecting a PCP is a major step in staying healthy. Do you have the right quarterback leading your health-care team?

The Rest of Your Health-Care Team

In addition to a PCP, you should consider adding a lifestyle medicine physician to your health-care team. According to the American College of Lifestyle Medicine website:

Lifestyle medicine is a medical specialty that uses therapeutic lifestyle interventions as a primary modality to treat chronic conditions including, but not limited to, cardiovascular diseases, type 2 diabetes, and obesity.

Lifestyle medicine certified clinicians are trained to apply evidence-based, whole-person, prescriptive lifestyle changes to treat and, when used intensively, often reverse such conditions.

Applying the six pillars of lifestyle medicine—a whole-food, plant-predominant eating pattern, physical activity, restorative sleep, stress management, avoidance of risky substances, and positive social connections—also provides effective prevention for these conditions.[5]

Lifestyle Medicine is not a curriculum in most medical schools. But the concept is becoming popular, and more physicians are getting board-certified in this practice.

Benefits of Wellness Coaching

Continuing with the team analogy, you've got your PCP as a quarterback and other members of your health-care team, so what about a coach?

Wellness is a multi-dimensional, comprehensive approach to enhancing a person's state of general well-being. It is about proactive intention, evolving toward a state of sustained wellness.

Wellness Continuum

	Poor Health	Neutral	Optimal State of Well-being
	Medical Paradigm		**Wellness Paradigm**
Reactive	Feel better		Thrive	Proactive
	Treat & cure illness		Maintain & improve health	
	Corrective		Preventive	
	Episodic		Holistic	
	Clinical responsibility		Individual responsibility	
	Compartmentalized		Integrated into life	

Source: Global Wellness Institute, adapted from Dr. Jack Travis

There are eight dimensions of wellness:

- **Physical:** a healthy body, achieved through nutrition, movement, and rest.
- **Mental:** intellectual engagement and a growth mindset that promotes learning.
- **Social:** a sense of connection with a community.
- **Relational:** deep intimacy with our loved ones.
- **Occupational:** a vibrant and fulfilling career.
- **Financial:** financial security.
- **Emotional:** being in touch with one's emotions and openly expressing them in a constructive manner.
- **Spiritual:** finding purpose and meaning in one's life.

Wellness is about paying close attention to all dimensions and ensuring that each supports the other. Being unwell in any dimension can permeate across the other dimensions, whereas achieving wellness across all dimensions promotes a greater sense of contentment and happiness.

In addition to these dimensions, there are internal (your beliefs, values, strengths, and attitudes) and external (your environment) forces at work that can either support or undermine your wellness.

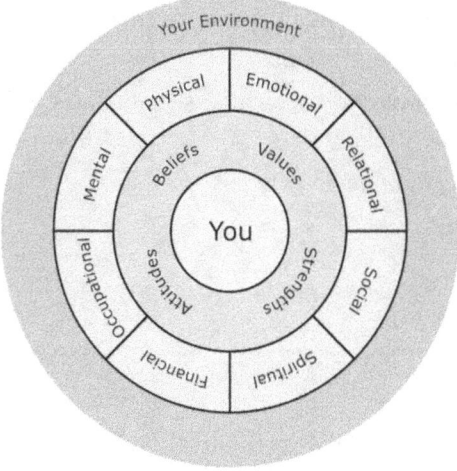

A good wellness coach can help you take inventory of these dimensions and factors and help you gain clarity around where you are, where you want to go, and how to focus your time and energy to get there. They will do this by getting to know you, your model of the world, your strengths, and your challenges. This enables them to collaborate with you to help you define and achieve your goals, tailoring solutions to your unique set of circumstances. They provide accountability to help you remain motivated and emotional support when times get tough and you encounter those inevitable roadblocks.

Track Your Health and Take Control

One simple way to keep track of your health is with a three-ring binder. You can get dividers (ones you can customize) and a good three-hole punch anywhere you get office supplies. Ask your doctors for copies of the appointment notes for each visit, copies of tests, etc. and store them in the binder. The following categories could be used for the dividers as methods to track your health:

- Schedule of checkups and tests
- List of prescriptions and supplements and the pharmacy you use
- Your healthcare team (business cards)
- Primary care physician—put all your correspondence with him/her here
- Copies of bloodwork and results
- List of immunizations and vaccinations (with dates when given)
- Copies of biopsies
- Copies of X-rays & bone density tests
- CDs of ultrasounds
- Bones
- Breasts (women)
- Colon
- Eyes
- Feet
- Skin

- Uterus and ovaries (women)
- Prostate (men)
- Teeth

Feel free to add other areas you want to keep track of or remove the ones you don't need. This is one of the best strategies to take control of your health. Health-care providers will be amazed when you take the binder to an appointment and can answer all their questions by quickly referring to it!

Do you have a complete health-care team you feel confident in? Take the time to make sure you have a health-care team that works for you for the long term. It is well worth the effort.

CHAPTER 3

Your Emotional and Mental Life

We become what we believe. So, we need to start by understanding what we think and believe before we can change our health. Our attitude plays a big part in our thriving or declining.

You first need to decide that *you deserve to be healthy* and understand what is stopping you. Otherwise, you won't make the changes to enable you to get there.

What beliefs need to be changed to make this happen?

By the time we reach our forties, we have experienced enough of life to have a basic idea of the changes that we need to make to be healthy. But most of us are so busy managing our life situations (job, career, caretaking, family, etc.) that we don't or haven't stopped to focus on our lives to make sure all is working well with us. And this kind of understanding doesn't happen without taking the time to step back and reflect.

The idea of taking this time for yourself may cause you to feel guilty or selfish, but nothing could be further from the truth. If you've ever taken a flight anywhere, you may recall that the flight crew always instructs you to put your own oxygen mask on first before helping others. That's because, if you're not right, you can't be there for those around you who need you. So, give yourself permission to take this time and think about what you need for yourself.

Intuitive Wisdom

After living for nearly half a century, we have curated much wisdom. And wisdom is part of our inner knowing. You have to decide that health is going to be a priority in your life. And you need to determine that you're going to do what you need to do to get healthy. Otherwise, it isn't going to happen. *It is your responsibility not anyone else's.* This may very well be the hardest of all the steps for you. This is not uncommon. As a result, you can read about being healthy but never take real action to achieve it, so you don't get anywhere.

We already know what we need to do and what we need to stop doing. The gift of our intuition needs to be included in this discussion. Gavin De Becker's book *The Gift of Fear* presents a convincing argument that you need to pay attention to your gut reactions, even if you can't exactly explain why. Listen carefully to your body and develop an appreciation for your intuitive way of knowing.

Brené Brown, a researcher known for her work on shame and vulnerability, explains how intuition works: "Intuition is not independent of any reasoning process. . . . [In fact,] psychologists believe that intuition is a rapid-fire, unconscious associating process, like a mental puzzle. The brain makes an observation, scans the files, and matches the observation with existing memories, knowledge, and experiences. Once it puts together a series of matches, we get a 'gut' on what we've observed."[1]

So don't ignore what your body (or intuition) is telling you about the changes that need to be made. But don't beat yourself up for whatever your situation is. Accept that you are where you are and move forward from there by taking action today.

Shaming and blaming aren't motivators. "Whatever your circumstances, research shows that long-term healthy habits aren't likely to result from fear, guilt, or shame. The motivation to do things that are good for your body and brain—and to make those good things into habits—comes from a positive place,"[2] shares Stephen Kopecky, MD.

And he should know! Dr. Kopecky is a cardiologist at the Mayo Clinic and a two-time cancer survivor. Fighting his second cancer led him to learn things he could do to prevent future cancer and major illness. Kopecky wanted to have the best health for as long as possible for the rest of his life. While he admits disease prevention was a new area for him, it led him to a different type of practice: the prevention side of medicine, which he works in today.[3]

Designing a Thriving Life

We get to where we are going by design or by default. By intention or accident. Our health is something many of us take for granted. So, we have health by default. And we don't think about it until . . . a problem appears. Then, when your health becomes an issue, you probably aren't very happy or thriving.

Thoughtful people since the beginning of humanity have understood that it pays to be healthy, say Bill Burnett and Dave Evans, authors of *Designing Your Life, How to Build a Well-Lived, Joyful Life*. Health is one of the four areas that fit in a life-design plan. Work, play, and love are the other three parts. Health is the foundation upon which work, play, and love stand. Without health, you can't have the other three.

A well-designed life is a generative life—it is constantly creative, productive, changing, and evolving. And there is always the possibility of surprise, share Burnett and Evans.[4] A well-designed life is at the core of aging gracefully. This book is rooted in this concept.

Small Habits Make Big Changes

Want to know how to make those healthy changes in your life? Start small. According to BJ Fogg, a PhD behavioral scientist at Stanford, many people fail at making lifestyle changes because it seems overwhelming. So, they never start, or they start too big and get discouraged by a lack of progress.

There are three things that you need to do to create successful habits so you can change your behaviors:

- Don't judge yourself.
- Focus on your aspirations and divide them into small actions.
- Think of mistakes as discoveries and use them to propel you forward.

This system removes the negative mindset that gets in your way. Instead, you learn to view behavior through the lens of a scientific experiment, where you explore and discover your way forward.

Growth Mindset

A growth mindset is a must for a healthy, thriving lifestyle. Good health is the result of the many small choices we make every day as a consequence of a well-designed routine. Will Bulsiewicz, MD, MSCI, a gastroenterologist, suggests that it is "when you build the right routine, then healing just happens. You're living a life that heals, restores, and strengthens you. And it's effortless. But to get there, we have to get into the right frame of mind." He practices a "health mindset."[5]

To develop new skills and change your life, Bulsiewicz advocates having a "growth mindset." A growth mindset is about what we are capable of becoming. Carol Dweck, PhD, pioneered the concept in her groundbreaking book *Mindset: The New Psychology of Success*.

Dweck, a world-class Stanford psychologist, researched how success in all areas is influenced by how we think about our talents. People with a growth mindset believe their abilities can be developed. Those with a fixed mindset believe their abilities are fixed, and they are therefore less likely to succeed than those with a growth mindset. This is important to remember as we age. Our abilities can improve, and aging should be about growing in all areas of our lives.

"The passion for stretching yourself and sticking to it, even (or especially) when it's not going well, is the hallmark of a growth mindset. This is the mindset that allows people to thrive during some of the most challenging times in their lives,"[6] states Dweck. Having a growth mindset can help you overcome many challenges as you make changes.

Ways to Manage Stress

In today's world, it is hard to manage stress. But we need to because it greatly affects our emotional and mental life. Stress is connected to six main causes of death—heart disease, cancer, lung issues, accidents, cirrhosis of the liver, and suicide[7]—explains Anne Ornish.

While we can't always change what happens to us, we can change our reactions.

The five different stress techniques that are explained in step-by-step instructions in the Ornishes *Undo It!* are:

- Gentle stretching
- Breathing techniques
- Meditation
- Guided imagery
- Deep relaxation[8]

Dr. Dean Ornish is the clinical professor of medicine at the University of California, San Francisco and founder and president of the Preventative Medicine Research Institute. Anne Ornish is the program director at the Preventative Medicine Research Institute.

You might want to try different techniques to see what works best for you. Many recommend finding one that works for you and sticking to it. You may find, for example, that daily meditation helps with achieving quality sleep and dealing with stress.

So have fun and experiment! The more you practice meditation or other stress-reduction techniques, the more you will feel the benefits.

Attitude of Gratitude

There is plenty of evidence that practicing gratitude frequently helps to make you healthier.[9] People who practice gratitude regularly are healthier and happier than those who don't.[10]

"One study even found that higher levels of gratitude resulted in better sleep. Results show that grateful people sleep better because they worry less and have fewer negative thoughts before falling asleep. They also tend to focus on positive things before falling asleep, which protects the quality of your sleep,"[11] shares Kopecky.

Because stress-reducing activities are good for your gut, Bulsiewicz recommends a simple meditation technique that integrates gratitude. Start with five minutes a day with these four steps:

- *Think of something you're grateful for. Focus on a positive thing that has happened to you.*
- *Think of someone you love. Take a moment to appreciate the positive role they have in your life.*
- *Clarify your intention. You're drawing a map to where you want to go. What do you want to happen in your life? This can be anything—an emotion, behavior, or goal. Make sure it's positive and something immediately applicable in the short term.*
- *Release your mind, focus on your breathing, and allow thoughts to naturally enter your mind. End with a few deep breaths and focus your eyes softly.*[12]

If you are feeling frustrated adjusting to the new normal and the fact that ambiguity is a part of it, try to remember to go to a place of gratitude. What are you grateful for? Sometimes, it is as simple as the fact that you're still breathing or you have a roof over your head. You may soon discover that staying with the feeling of frustration usually doesn't serve you well. So go to gratitude!

Life will always present challenges that we will need to overcome. Practicing gratitude is part of overcoming those challenges. And there is always a lesson. Life is telling you something that you need to pay attention to. Try to learn the lesson early, and life works out better. Learning early saves some pain, which is something else you can be grateful for!

The Power of Resilience

Resilience is another quality to cultivate in your life. In her TED talk, Lucy Hone shares the three strategies that resilient people use to navigate through tough times:

- Know that bad things happen and suffering is normal.
- Choose carefully what you focus on. Put your attention on what is in your power to change and accept the things you can't. Asking what is in your control gives you back power and lets you focus on what you can control. Find things to be grateful for.
- Ask yourself if the way you are thinking or acting is helping you or hurting you. Then choose to release the things that are hurting you.[13]

Restorative Sleep

Sleep is critical to good health. Hence, we need to make it a priority. Most adults need seven to nine hours of sleep a night. Are you getting that?

Sleep deprivation has been called a public health epidemic.

"Sleep is an essential function that allows your body and mind to recharge, leaving you refreshed and alert when you wake up." Healthy sleep helps to keep your body healthy and helps to keep you from getting diseases.[14] And during sleep, our immunity is increased as our body makes cytokines, a type of protein that targets infection and inflammation and are messengers for our immune system, according to SleepFoundation.org.[15]

When sleep is a problem, it is time to pay attention! "It's a clue that something about your lifestyle is asking to be adjusted, or something else in your body needs attention,"[16] suggests Dr. Frank Lipman. He also recommends that a pharmaceutical sleep aid *not* be used, as it has been proven to increase dementia risk, is addictive, and can cause strange behaviors.[17] Lipman is a pioneer in both integrative and functional medicine.

How can you set yourself up for a good night's sleep? Lipman suggests the following secrets from successful sleepers:

- *Go to bed when you are tired*
- *Don't eat your evening meals too late*
- *Avoid alcohol close to bedtime*
- *Leave technology (and TV) out of the bedroom*
- *Have the WI-FI router on a timer*
- *Sleep in a very dark room*
- *Stay comfortably cool at night*
- *Work out the necessary changes with your partner*
- *Use an alternative alarm clock*
- *Don't go to bed angry*[18]

The bottom line is that the sleep period is critical to our health and emotional and mental well-being. And don't be afraid to get help to achieve quality sleep if you need it.

Keep Building Your Brain & Increase Your Cognitive Reserve with Lifelong Learning

"There is no cure for Alzheimer's disease once it has manifested, but you can be cognitively active, reverse debilitating symptoms, and add happy healthy years to your life even with an Alzheimer's diagnosis. Lifestyle matters,"[19] state Drs. Ayesha and Dean Sherzai. "Alzheimer's develops decades before a diagnosis. It's during those decades that the brain becomes increasingly vulnerable to what we eat, how much we exercise, our ability to manage chronic stress, the quality of our sleep, and the ways we challenge our cognitive abilities. Only later on, often when we reach our sixties and seventies, is the brain unable to compensate for our less than healthy choices, and that's when we first begin to notice changes in thinking and memory,"[20] advise the Sherzais.

Besides living a healthy lifestyle, the Sherzais say that we need to participate in complex activities by challenging multiple functions in the brain. A few examples they recommend include:

- *Learning a new language*
- *Learning a musical instrument*
- *Computer programming*
- *Writing a book*
- *Karaoke and singing*
- *Performing stand-up comedy*
- *Learning to dance*
- *Chess club or group card games (bridge, gin, rummy, poker, etc.)*
- *Mentoring others in your field*
- *Volunteering to teach children math, English, or any subject you enjoy*
- *Jewelry, crafts, models, or art*
- *Taking community college courses*[21]

Do you see any activities you might want to try?

Do You Play?

Brené Brown says, "I now understand that play is as essential to our health and functioning as rest."[22]

Have you ever thought about the importance that play holds in our lives as adults?

"A lack of play should be treated as malnutrition—it's a health risk to your body and soul,"[23] says Stuart Brown, MD. Dr. Brown is a medical doctor, psychiatrist, clinical researcher, and founder of the National Institute for Play.

Play isn't something we need to do all the time to be fulfilled, but it can serve as a catalyst. "The beneficial effects of getting just a little true play can spread through our lives, actually making us more productive and happier in everything we do,"[24] suggests Brown.

Brown shares a story:

> One example of this is Laurel, the CEO of a successful commercial real estate company. During her late twenties, Laurel married and had two children, all while establishing her business. Her relationship with her husband was close and compatible, and she adored her four and ten-year-olds. She saw herself as blessed and fortunate.
>
> Her days hummed like a turbocharged engine. Up at five, she usually ran four or five miles on odd days and swam and lifted weights on even days. She didn't work weekends and usually had enough steam left for 'quality time' with her supportive husband and kids, church, and closest friends.
>
> She felt she had a healthy mix of play and work, but when she passed forty, she began to dread her schedule. She didn't yet feel a need to quit any of her commitments or ease off, but slowly she realized that though she had fun with her husband and kids and a sense of enthusiasm about her work, she was missing . . . joy.
>
> So Laurel set about finding where it had gone. She remembered back to her earliest joyful memories and realized they centered on horses.

As a young adult who competed as a professional rider, she eventually left horse shows and settled into marriage and business.

Yet she now realized she longed 'just to ride.'

Laurel decided to make this happen. She found a horse to lease and began to ride again. The feelings of joy and exhilaration came back the first time she climbed on a horse. Now, she makes time to go riding once a week.

What surprises her most since she incorporated the pure play of riding back into her life is how whole she now feels in all other areas of her life. The bloom of 'irrational bliss' she experiences in the care of her horse, from riding it regularly and even occasionally riding again in small horse shows, has spilled over into her family and work lives. The little chores of daily living don't seem so difficult anymore.[25]

There is a magical quality in play. "Once people understand what play does for them, they can learn to bring a sense of excitement and adventure back to their lives, make work an extension of their play lives, and engage fully in the world,"[26] concludes Brown.

Consider the positive impact that play can have on your own health. Where can you invest some of your time? You may be surprised at how "playtime" feeds your soul and helps to contribute to an overall sense of joy and happiness.

So, what exactly constitutes play? Brown says there are seven characteristics of healthy play:

1. *Apparently purposeless (done for its own sake)*
2. *Voluntary*
3. *Inherent attraction*
4. *Freedom from time*
5. *Diminished consciousness of self*
6. *Improvisational potential*
7. *Continuation desire*[27]

"Play is about joy . . . play is any activity that brings you joy when you do it,"[28] state Burnett and Evans. Play can be an organized activity or competitive experience when done for the joy and delight in doing them. "When an activity is done to win, to advance, to achieve—even if it's 'fun' to do so—it's not play."[29]

Importance of Connections and Engagement

We are hardwired to be with and around people. The power of connection does wonders for our emotional health.

"The need for authentic connection and community is primal, as fundamental to our health and well-being as the need for air, water, and food,"[30] says Dr. Dean Ornish. There are thousands of studies "showing that people who feel lonely, depressed, and irritated are three to ten times more likely to get sick and die prematurely from virtually all causes when compared to those who have strong feelings of love, connection, and community."[31]

So make sure you have a support system consisting of people that really help the actions you are taking to get healthy. Yes, if you fall off the wagon, you might need assistance getting back on. Don't be afraid to get it. Supportive people are huge for our emotional health. You can find some in the Resource section of this book. There is an abundance of help out there.

What Can We Do When Our Network Isn't Supportive?

While family and friends can be our biggest gifts, they can also be our biggest challenges.

Some people have a hard time accepting us when we start making changes in our lives. And because we want to fit in, we go back to our unhealthy habits. This doesn't help us move forward on our path so we can be healthy and thrive.

Instead, like crabs in a bucket, we are stopped by others. When crabs are in a bucket, the minute one crab tries to climb out of it, another crab will start physically pulling it back down with the rest. People can do the same thing.

Instead, it is important to stay focused and not let others deter you from making the changes that will help you be healthy. Here are some suggestions that can help you stay motivated:

- **Stay on your path.** Yes, it is easy to get detoured by criticism. Instead, continue and be persistent. And don't give up! Take it one day at a time.
- **Invite naysayers to join you.** Share your knowledge and help them grow too. Maybe the person criticizing you feels left out.
- **Seek help if you are stuck.** If you need assistance with something, don't be afraid to reach out. Many people want to help others (or know others that can help) and just might have the solution you need to move forward.
- **Connect with people already living a healthy, thriving lifestyle.** Many people living this way would be thrilled that you reached out to them. So don't be shy about asking. Seek others that support growth and a healthy lifestyle. As the saying goes, you are the company you keep.

With the limited years that you have left on this earth, how do you want to spend your time? Managing chronic disease or terminal illness? Or living life, thriving?

Feeling Stuck?

There's a lot to consider here. And it can feel overwhelming. What can you do if you are overwhelmed? What can you do if you're motivated to make some of these changes but have no idea where to start? What if you're feeling unmotivated? Or you lack vision for where you want to go? How do you move forward? How do you make progress?

There is a simple solution, and it's only two words: *do something.*

This is a simple yet very powerful thing to remember. Here are some reasons to get yourself unstuck by doing something:

- **Doing something is better than doing nothing.** The most basic reason for doing something is that it's better than doing nothing. If you're feeling overwhelmed and are paralyzed by it and take no action, then you will simply not make any progress in anything. If, however, you choose one single action, no matter how small, it is a step in the right direction. Remember the old adage, "A journey of a thousand miles begins with a single step." The only way to accomplish big things is through the compounding of small efforts.

- **It can give you clarity.** You might be tempted to wait to do something until you have complete clarity around what it is you want to accomplish. It's natural to want to define a goal and then put a plan in place. But if you don't feel completely certain about what you're trying to accomplish, how will you get that clarity? By simply doing something, you will get feedback from it. Either it felt good and you enjoyed it and now you have something to build upon or you didn't get anything out of it, in which case you simply (and this is a little more complex because it's three words) **do something else**. Doing something gives you the gift of an actual experience, which is much more valuable than sitting around imagining how doing something might feel.

- **Small commitments can lead to greater effort.** To overcome resistance, commit to doing something very small. You may find that, once you do that small thing, it gives you energy to continue naturally. For example, you know you should go to the gym, but you're not feeling up to it. Commit to going to the gym and doing five minutes on the treadmill or a single weight machine, whatever you like to do at the gym. Chances are you'll continue beyond that initial commitment. And if not, that's fine. At least you did something. Which we already know is better than doing nothing.

- **You can interrupt a vicious cycle.** There are two types of cycles we can get ourselves into. The vicious cycle and the virtuous cycle. The vicious cycle is fed by negativity. It's the cycle that looks at how far you are from something you want to accomplish, tells you that you can't do it, it's too hard, and then as time passes, your inaction confirms it, perhaps pushing you even farther away from where you want to go. Simply doing something can interrupt this process, giving you a sense of accomplishment and setting you on a virtuous cycle.

  A virtuous cycle is one fed by positivity, where you clearly see the results of your efforts, getting you closer to where you want to go and generating a natural motivation to continue. The results begin to compound, making further efforts seem . . . effortless.

- **You can overcome the fear of failure.** Inaction due to a fear of failure is your brain's way of keeping you safe. It takes on the form of procrastination and "analysis paralysis." Procrastination happens because the safest way to avoid failure is to simply avoid action. You can't fail if you don't try. Analysis paralysis arises when you seek more information and over-thinking your next step. Your brain is trying to get a guarantee that you will succeed before even trying. Since no such guarantees exist, your brain is never satisfied enough to let you get started. Your fear of failure must be met head-on by just doing something and seeing what happens. Remember the growth mindset. Failure is a necessary part of learning.

Now that we have given you many areas of your emotional and mental health to consider, what is stopping you from being healthy?

CHAPTER 4

So Why Do You Want to Live Longer?

Why are you reading this book? Why do you care about your health? Why are you here on this planet? What matters to you most? What's next? It's fair to assume that you are reading this book because you want to live the best, longest life you can. You will need to make changes to accomplish this. And let's face it: change is hard! So these are the critical questions you need to ask yourself. Your answers will help you envision the future you want for yourself. Write down a vision for yourself and post it where you will see it multiple times a day. Connect emotionally with that vision. Feel it. Make it central to your decision-making process.

"I believe every one of us is born with a purpose. No matter who you are, what you do, or how far you think you have to go, you have been tapped by a force greater than yourself to step into your God-given calling. This goes far beyond what you do to earn your living. I'm talking about a supreme moment of destiny, the reason you are here on earth,"[1] states Oprah Winfrey.

Abraham Maslow believed that we have an inner knowing that encourages us to live up to our full potential and "grow healthy, fruitful, and happy." If denied or suppressed, the lack of expression of the inner nature, he argued, "leads to sickness,"[2] says Michael Arloski, PhD, PCC, CWP. Maslow is credited with developing the self-actualization theory. Arloski is the author of *Wellness Coaching for Lasting Lifestyle Change*.

"Knowing what you want out of life can be a great motivator. So, once you understand your meaning and purpose, use that as an inspiration to live your best life,"[3] shares Kopecky.

Only you know for sure what gives your life meaning. But how can you find it if you don't know what you want? Spend some quiet time and consider Lipman's and Kopecky's suggestions below.

According to Lipman, your purpose is not something you discover. "Instead, it comes from following your passions and interests, and spending time on the small things that are important to you."[4]

Also, Kopecky recommends spending time answering the following questions to help you uncover your "why" to find your purpose:

- *What activities make me feel excited, fulfilled, or rewarded?*
- *When do I feel like the best version of me?*
- *What are my natural gifts, talents, and abilities?*
- *How do I best help others?*
- *What three (or five or seven) ideas, actions, or events are important to me?*
- *What have I always wanted to try?*
- *What activities do I most look forward to each day, week, or month?*
- *What have I been putting off until I have more time?*
- *What relationships are important to me?*
- *Are there relationships that I'd like to make stronger or invest more time in?*
- *What do I want my days to look like? What about my weeks and years?*
- *Does it feel like something is missing from my life? What is it?*
- *If I could do anything, what would that be?*[5]

Rekindling an Old Passion

Suzanne Watkins figured out she needed a job in travel while participating in a transformational workshop at the Modern Elder Academy (MEA) in February 2018. Earlier in 2018, she had a life-threatening sepsis infection that required half of her intestine to be removed. According to an article in The Guardian, she said, "It made me realize that I'm mortal. Sometimes that's what it takes."[6]

While recovering at home, she began to see life from a different angle. Suzanne didn't want to return to her office job. Instead, she wanted to explore the world and decided she could do that as a flight attendant and get paid to do it.

As a result, she downsized her life and put her belongings in a storage unit. Suzanne's love for *National Geographic* magazines, drawing pictures of airplanes, and requesting brochures from faraway places was finally realized. Before her illness, she says, "I was complacent. And complacency and old age—it doesn't work. It's not uplifting. I think it's important as an older adult to keep pushing limits. . . . Think of it as continuing to unfold. And you can have surprises and joy."[7]

Same Job, Different Attitudes

Ornish shares another way to look at the importance of one's purpose or "why" in the old story of three stone cutters:

> *The first one complains, "Can't see what I'm doing? I'm cutting stones into blocks, and I will be doing this until the day I die."*
>
> *The second one, "I'm earning a living so I can support my beloved family. I can provide clothing and food in our home filled with love."*
>
> *The third one proclaims joyfully, "I have the privilege to help build a great cathedral so magnificent it will inspire people and lift their spirits for a thousand years!"*[8]

So, what's yours? Why do you want to live longer? And healthier in the process? Now is the time to get clear about what a thriving, healthy life looks like for you. Ask yourself what you want to be in the world. **Write it down. Be curious.** What's left to still do?

Help Fix the Planet

We can't discuss our health without bringing up our planet's health. In closing this chapter, you are encouraged to look around at what's going on in the world. And see if there is something you can do to help fix some of the problems that plague us today. A few to consider:

- The health of the planet
- Global warming
- The state of our health
- The alarming number of species disappearing

Yes, don't be afraid to try. Please don't just sit on the sidelines and do nothing to help if you have ideas. You have enormous wisdom, life experience, and skills. And your gift of action (small or large) could create a tipping point to help solve so much of what is broken today. And that shouldn't be wasted.

To be honest, the condition of the planet that we are handing to the next generations is quite alarming. That is one of the motivations for writing this book. So, if you see a problem, do what you can to help. That is a good reason to want to live longer. We are striving to show women and men numerous ways to take control of their health so they can live their longest lives, thriving, and in the process, help heal the planet.

Quality of Life

It is an undeniable fact that we are all going to die sometime. Some of us will go quickly, unexpectedly. Some of us will be fortunate enough to live a much longer life. But what good is a longer life if it is fraught with significant health issues that prevent us from doing what we want to do? Or even worse, preventing us from enjoying our own existence?

Regardless of whether you are in perfect health now or have some lingering issues, the time to take control of your health is now. Not tomorrow. Not next week. Not waiting for the next set of New Year's resolutions to come and go. Right now!

There's a trajectory that your health is currently on, and you possess the ability to change that trajectory. Take a look at this chart from "A global strategy for healthy ageing"[9] by Kalache and Kickbusch, published in *World Health*, 1997.

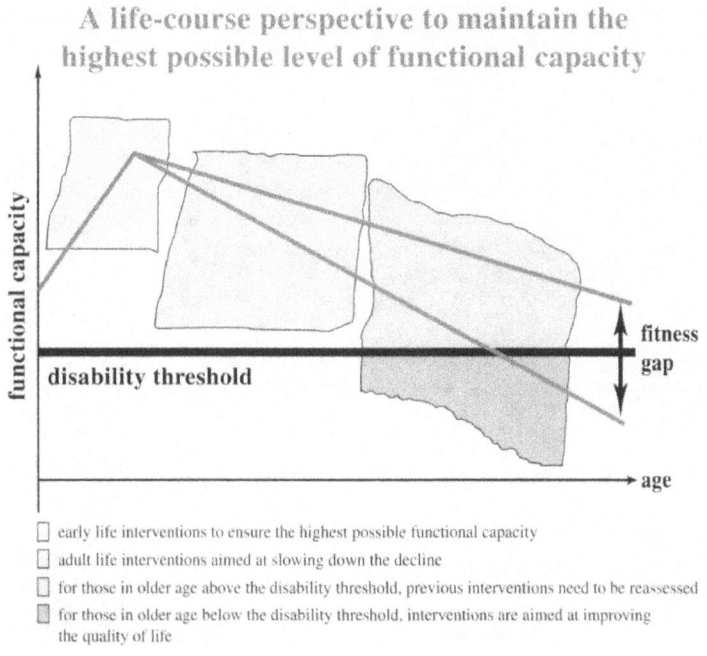

The "fitness gap" depicted above is under *your direct influence*. Whether you track on the top line or the bottom line or somewhere in between will be largely dictated by the choices you make today, tomorrow, and for the rest of your life.

Before moving on, take some time to think about *why you want to live longer*.

Next, we will discuss taking your first steps toward living a healthier, longer life.

CHAPTER 5

Your Nutritional Life

Let food be your medicine, and medicine be your food.

—Hippocrates

Your diet is the foundation for being healthy. "Diet is the top risk factor for disease and early death worldwide . . . [and] also has a profound effect on aging and increases the risk of diseases such as cancer and diabetes,"[1] explains Kopecky.

Did you know that 70% of our immune system lives in our gut? In fact, Bulsiewicz thinks that "[a]ll health and disease start in the gut."[2]

Analyzing your nutritional life can be a pivotal point for you. You can continue to put food that is damaging your health into your body, or you can give your body food that nourishes it. The *decision* is yours and yours alone. No amount of advice or knowledge gathering will make a difference. Only informed changes will lead to the results you're pursuing.

But what is a good diet today?

Four Dietary Patterns Associated with Reducing Chronic Disease Today

Four established dietary patterns stand out that dieticians, nutritionists, and functional or lifestyle physicians recommend and are heavily studied, shares Gigi Carter, a licensed nutritionist. While all diets are similar in that they consist of whole-plant foods, they differ.

They are:

- *Whole-Food, Plant-Based (WFPB)—entirely plant-based*
- *Vegan—entirely plant-based*
- *The Ornish Diet—Low-fat, high in complex carbohydrates, and almost entirely plant-based with a few animal-based exceptions*
- *Mediterranean Diet and the DASH diet—More plant-based than the typical Western-style diet but also comprise moderate portions of various animal products in lean forms*

"All four of these dietary patterns have been associated with reducing chronic disease risk, and those that are more plant-based produce the best outcomes for reducing and even reversing chronic diseases,"[3] continues Carter. More about Carter can be found in Chapters 6 and 7.

What Is a Whole Food, Plant-Based (WFPB) Diet?

A WFPB diet that has been proven to reverse the progression of many different chronic diseases, according to Dr. Dean Ornish, includes:

- *Consume mostly plants ("good carbs" and "good protein"): vegetables, fruits, whole grains, legumes, soy products, and small amounts of nuts and seeds in forms as close as possible to their natural, unprocessed state.*
- *What you include in your diet is as important as what you exclude. There are thousands of protective factors in plant-based foods that have anticancer,*

anti-heart disease, and antiaging properties as well as being very low in disease-promoting substances.
- Minimize or, even better, eliminate animal protein and replace it with plant-based protein.
- Avoid sugar, white flour, white rice, and other "bad carbs."
- Consume 3 grams per day of "good fats" (omega-3 fatty acids).
- Reduce intake of total fat, and especially "bad fats," such as trans fats, saturated fats, and partially hydrogenated fats.
- Organic is optimal—foods taste much better; and they are much lower in pesticide residues, which can disrupt your hormones.[4]

Furthermore, Dr. T. Colin Campbell explains, "At its simplest and most accessible, the WFPB diet can be described in a dozen words, distilled in two recommendations:
- Consume a variety of whole, plant-based foods.
- Avoid consumption of animal-based foods."[5]

Campbell continues, "A WFPB diet is not the same thing as a vegan diet, which is defined by:

> What it eliminates: animal foods. A WFPB diet is defined also by what it emphasizes: A variety of whole-plant foods. By whole, I mean all [of] a food's nutrients are consumed together, regardless of whether the foods are diced, sliced, cooked, or blended. I also mean that added oils and refined carbohydrates, such as table sugar, should be used sparingly, if at all. So-called convenience foods like potato chips are not whole. High in refined ingredients, they undermine health in every respect; they are calorically replete, nutrient deficient, and absolutely inconvenient in the long term. (Or can you imagine a scenario in which sudden coronary death is convenient?)

> No diet has ever been shown to not only prevent but also reverse heart disease, and there exist no large-scale, international correlation studies that show the opposite effect (increased animal protein consumption associated with decreased heart disease, cancer, etc.). Moreover, there are virtually no nutrients contained in animal foods that are not better provided by plant foods.[6]

Dr. Campbell is responsible for the term whole food, plant-based. And he is the Jacob Gould Schurman Professor Emeritus of Nutritional Biochemistry in the Division of Nutritional Sciences at Cornell University and the co-author of *The China Study*. *The China Study* is the most comprehensive study of nutrition ever conducted and the surprising implications for diet, weight loss, and long-term health. And we are honored that he has written the Foreword on this book.

Can Food Prevent Alzheimer's Disease?

New hope exists for preventing Alzheimer's disease, the sixth leading cause of death! Ninety percent of the cases can be prevented, according to the Sherzais.[7] Nutritional food along with other lifestyle changes can prevent, reverse, and/or delay onset.

Deaths "due to Alzheimer's have increased by nearly 87% in the last decade,"[8] state the Sherzais. Food is the greatest tool we have to keep from getting Alzheimer's due to the fundamental role it plays in "sustaining and regulating the body," the doctors contend. They also say,

> As lifestyle physicians and researchers, we cannot overstate the importance of food for brain health; it is by far the most important lifestyle factor. The dietary choices we make every day influence the prevention, delay, or progression of cognitive decline. Our clinical research has shown again and again, with patients of all ages and degrees of neurodegenerative disease, that adhering to a brain-healthy diet results in better cognition. It's that simple.[9]

And a brain-healthy diet (as part of a healthy lifestyle) is a "whole-food, plant-based diet low in sugar, salt, and processed foods,"[10] explain the Sherzais.

WFPB Diet Put to the Test: The Power of Food Over COVID-19

In December 2021, a Harvard study confirmed that a healthy diet was connected with lower COVID-19 risk and severity.[11] Furthermore, the researchers noted that getting vaccinated and wearing a mask in indoor settings were also important tactics to keep from getting the virus.

Can a WFPB Diet Reverse Cancer?

Campbell shares that his wife was diagnosed with "stage III advanced melanoma, the most serious kind of skin cancer." She had the cancer tissue removed surgically, and the sentinel node of the lymph gland was biopsied. They found cancer had spread to the lymphatic system. And three pathologists agreed with the diagnosis.[12]

However, she decided she did not want to have additional surgery. Instead, she decided to do nothing but eat only plant-based foods. Eight years later, she "is in excellent health."

"I feel that Karen's diet not only helped her after the cancer diagnosis but in the years preceding it. . . . It is highly likely that this mole was cancerous prior to our family's conversion to a plant-based diet and that its progress was slowed or suspended, or perhaps even reversed, after this point. The results of the biopsy may even have shown cancer retreating rather than spreading,"[13] shares Campbell.

How to Learn to Cook WFPB Meals

While converting to a WFPB diet can be a game changer, it does have challenges. For most people, the hardest thing will be learning how to cook food all over again. And it needs to be easy to learn and simple to do, or many people will abandon the notion. But, most of all, it needs to taste good!

Here are some great books you can use to learn about the diet/lifestyle (no meat, no sugar, no oil, little or no processed foods, no dairy, and only legumes, vegetables, and fruit):

- *The Forks Over Knives Plan: How to Transition to the Life-Saving, Whole-Food, Plant-Based Diet*, by Alona Pulde, MD, and Matthew Lederman, MD
- *Forks Over Knives Cookbook*, by Del Sroufe
- *The Engine 2 Diet: The Texas Firefighter's 28-Day Save-Your-Life Plan that Lowers Cholesterol and Burns Away Pounds*, by Rip Esselstyn

This may be all you need to get yourself started. They have instructions on how to organize your kitchen and how to cook and lots of great recipes. Hopefully, you will find that transitioning to a WFPB diet can start very simply. The three books above do a great job of creating a foundation for learning this diet/lifestyle.

Now that you know what a healthy diet is and what a WFPB one can do for your health, let's go to the next chapter, where you'll meet four people practicing a WFPB lifestyle today.

CHAPTER 6

How and Why Others Started on the WFPB Path

Meet Rod Horn

Rod Horn had a 100% blockage of the left anterior descending artery (LAD) before he changed his diet and lifestyle. He has now completed several ultra-marathons with impressive results and feels great. He says,

I have been WFPB since 2019, for four glorious years. I started my WFPB journey a week or two after my heart attack and never looked back.

Previously, my wife, Amy, started having rheumatoid arthritis (RA) problems in her mid-forties. After doing some research, she approached me and asked what I thought about a vegan diet. I told her to go right ahead; I'm not interested. Unfortunately, she didn't follow through with the diet, and I was clueless about what my diet was doing to my body.

In my mid-forties, I began running to get more exercise. I carried extra weight, but I became a 5k runner. I had no clue what was to come.

As an active fifty-two-year-old, my widowmaker heart attack was not at all expected. My symptoms came about abruptly, and I felt hot, sweaty, and nauseous. Certainly not what was portrayed in the movies. I knew something was not right, so my son drove me to the hospital less than half a mile away. Luckily, my quick actions allowed me to receive a stent, returning the flow of blood to my heart and saving my life.

A good friend (a doctor) with heart disease in her family visited me in the hospital. When Amy told her we might make dietary changes, she shared

the benefits of a WFPB lifestyle with us. Our first instruction was to watch the Forks Over Knives movie. We watched it, and that began our WFPB journey.

My doctor friend shared the how and why of WFPB. So we emptied the house of all the food that should not be in our diet and started figuring things out. We worked very hard to eat healthy and made plenty of mistakes along the way. But we quickly established what food would become our new staples.

Horn considers himself WFPB, not vegan:

I am whole food, plant-based. The difference is that I attempt to eat foods that are plant-based and are as close to the source as possible. Another major difference is that I work extremely hard to stay away from oils and fats (which are permitted in a vegan diet). Because of my heart disease, I do not eat nuts and most seeds. In addition, I stay away from avocados and olives.

Before my heart attack, I was a pescatarian (eating fish and seafood with a vegetarian diet) and believed that was eating healthy. It was so far from the truth. I was a terrible pescatarian, like many vegans that eat highly processed foods today. I ate lots of highly processed fatty foods. Cheese was a daily favorite. Now, I understand the importance of reading food labels.

When asked who is successful at making this change, Horn said,

I have often discussed with my doctor friend what it takes to become WFPB. And I think that most people are unwilling to make the change because they are following what they believed their entire lives. Americans have been sold the story that the Standard American Diet (SAD) is fine, but they are totally unaware of the consequences. If you follow the money through marketing and advertisements, it is easy to see that we are encouraged to eat highly processed foods. When was the last time you saw a commercial for spinach, beans, or rice?

In discussing the difference that a WFPB lifestyle has made in his life and his family, Horn stated,

It has been an incredible journey these last four years.

I feel great! I didn't go into this trying to lose weight but lost forty pounds, and it only took six months. My little running hobby has exploded. Last year, I ran several ultramarathons. An ultramarathon is a distance greater than a marathon distance. My longest race to date was 37 miles. I ran a half marathon in Hawaii during my thirtieth anniversary and came in fifth overall, so my speed has increased tremendously.

My wife has controlled her diabetes with the diet, eliminating all medications and most RA symptoms. She also lost over forty pounds and kept it off.

For people that want to start but don't know how to begin, Horn suggests,

Nutritionsfacts.org is a wealth of information. Dr. Michael Greger provides the WFPB information for free. Jump in with both feet, knowing that you might make mistakes and that you will get smarter as you go. Be nice to yourself as you figure it out, but go for it and make it happen. Your life may depend on it!

Start today! Find others in your area that can support you and share ideas. Batch cook your food so you're not spending too much time preparing food.[1]

Meet Chris Kalinich

Chris Kalinich has been following a WFPB lifestyle since early 2015. She chose to ease herself and her family into healthier eating habits, eliminating ultra-processed foods, reducing meat and dairy, and cooking from scratch. "It all clicked for me when I attended a two-day immersion program to educate university employees about a research study led by a prominent plant-based physician. I realized I had nothing to lose and the potential to gain so much," shares Kalinich.

She followed the arrows pointing her toward a WFPB lifestyle. Like many of us, she tried various approaches to healing her body, but nothing worked. She says,

I made the change to the WFPB way of eating when I recognized that the ultra-processed and animal-based food on my plate was negatively impacting my health. I suffered from gall bladder issues, symptoms of IBS [irritable bowel syndrome], migraines, high cholesterol, and fatigue. Gut health is the driver of overall body and brain health.

I felt like I was educating myself so I could educate my doctors. I didn't want to apply Band-aids to my symptoms. I needed to understand the root causes of my issues so I could tackle them head-on to be rid of them. Functional nutrition understands that the body's systems are intricately complex and interconnected. The body flourishes in a state of balance, and our food choices can either support or harm this balance.

When I started to place healthier options on my plate, these issues began to quickly recede. The simple yet effective solution was to remove foods that were inflammatory to my body and introduce plant foods that were healing and promoted a healthy gut microbiome.

The results? I still have my gallbladder. I no longer suffer from digestive issues. Migraines are a thing of the past. I manage my lipids with plants and not medicine. And I am twenty pounds lighter than I was in my twenties, and my energy levels are great!

The experience led Kalinich to her purpose:

[As a result,] my goal is to help everyone experience the benefits of optimum nutrition by discovering joy in the kitchen and to enjoy life one flavorful bite at a time!

Food has always been a huge part of my life, and I think it is significant for most people. We connect with our food in many ways: physically, emotionally, biologically, chemically, and even spiritually. We often associate it with social occasions, family heritage, life experiences, and cultural identification. Food is a vital component of who we are.

When I discovered that food choice was the kingpin for many of the health issues I was suffering from, I decided to make it my life purpose to help others understand the connection between food and health outcomes. I am humbled and honored to work with so many diverse people who want to reclaim their lives and achieve their vision of wellness (breast cancer survivors, food pantry clients, those recovering from drug addiction, and retirees who refuse to retire!).

My background is in education and corporate training, and I love to facilitate the process for others to discover the best version of themselves, no matter where they are within their lifespan. I combine nutrition counseling and nutrition education with culinary coaching to help people fall in love again with their food ... in a healthy, nourishing way.

She has discovered that the people who are most successful transitioning into a WFPB diet understand that food is the solution, not the enemy, and they believe that they do control what they put on their plates. "Real food, WFPB food, nourishes the body, mind, and soul. None of us are perfect in anything that we do, and it is okay if we fail sometimes. Just pick up and move forward. Everyone is unique, and thus, the food journey for each person will be different," states Kalinich.

On overcoming resistance from family members: "I always think compassionate honesty is the best policy when it comes to communicating with family members. If one gently communicates the 'why' behind the decision, the change is more easily accepted," she shares. Also,

We must recognize that family and friends may question the change because they fear losing their loved one to a "fad diet" or feel judged that they eat differently. Asking for their support of the decision is not the same as requiring them to change with you. Everyone's health journey is unique.

If you feel the need for outside support, most communities have plant-based outreach organizations. The Google Search engine is a great way to find like-minded support groups and fun meetups.

For people who are wanting to start but don't know how to focus on the "why" question, Kalinich recommends they ask themselves if they want to be able to:

- *Get down on the floor and play with my kids or grandkids?*
- *Backpack the Grand Canyon?*
- *Be free of pain and the fear that my body is working against me?*
- *Dance with unbridled joy with my partner?*

Whatever your "why," keep that in mind as you make the change. Be your authentic self with a passion! Don't worry about how fast you make the change or what others are thinking. Instead, approach each day with intention and take an actionable step to get you to your best self.

"The decision to eat WFPB has impacted my life in so many positive ways. As I improved how I ate and saw the beneficial results, I made other lifestyle changes. I had the energy to become more physically active, so I am now a huge outdoor enthusiast. Being mindful of my food choices directed me to be more mindful in other aspects of my life: relationships, quality of sleep, exercise, and stress management. WFPB is not just a way of eating; it is a holistic lifestyle that promotes vitality,"[2] concludes Kalinich.

Meet Amanda Strombom

In 1996, Strombom was living in Malaysia and getting sick, on occasion, from eating unrefrigerated meat that had been prepared and served from market stalls. Encouraged by some friends who were vegetarians, Strombom decided to give it a try.

When she moved to the US in 1997, she volunteered to help a vegetarian organization holding an annual food festival. Soon, she was leading the organization and subsequently went on to form a new organization. During that experience, she learned about the health benefits of eating plants, the environmental benefits, and the benefits for animals. That information made her even more committed to this lifestyle.

Today, Strombom reports,

> My husband and I are now in our sixties and very healthy. I have no medical conditions. My husband has high blood pressure, which seems to be related to stress and anxiety. However, he is very healthy apart from that. It's hard to know how our health would have been if we had not changed our diet so many years ago, but we're very glad that we made the switch.
>
> I saw the benefits of going vegan right away but found that my husband and children weren't ready to go from vegetarian to vegan in the early days. I

introduced them to various dairy substitutes and minimized the use of dairy and eggs to the extent I could until my children left home. At that point, it became much easier for my husband and myself to be fully vegan. The available dairy substitutes these days would likely have made this an easier process.

In 2014, I took the Physician's Committee for Responsible Medicine's training to be a Food for Life cooking instructor. This was my introduction to the concept of a WFPB diet. I now consider myself to be largely WFPB. The definition I prefer to use is that a vegan diet avoids all animal products but allows for junk food that may be high in processed foods, sugar, salt, and oil. In contrast, a WFPB diet, in addition to avoiding all animal products, minimizes or totally avoids overly processed foods and sugar, salt, and oil. I use sugar, salt, and oil very sparingly, though I still love a little dark chocolate from time to time.

Strombom has found the people most successful at making this change in diet are those who suffer from chronic diseases such as:

Type 2 diabetes, heart disease, Crohn's disease, and rheumatoid arthritis, to name just a few. When they discover or ideally are told by their doctor that they need to change to a WFPB diet to avoid the disease getting any worse, they often feel like their health is in danger if they don't make the change. So, many are highly motivated to change their diet almost overnight.

Unfortunately, far too few doctors are aware of the power of a plant-based diet to prevent and treat many diseases, and they don't feel confident in prescribing a plant-based diet to their patients. This means that many patients with chronic diseases who could be helped by a WFPB diet are not given the advice and support they need.

People who learn about the impact of animal agriculture on the animals themselves and hold the welfare of animals as one of their most important values are also highly motivated to avoid animal products.

To begin eating this way, Strombom says,

I would suggest that trying out some meat substitute products and using them to replace meat in favorite dishes is a good place to start. While these foods are processed, they are much healthier than meat and can be very useful in

[the] transition. Similarly, replacing any animal-based staples, such as cow's milk, cheese, and ice cream with dairy substitutes based on nuts or grains, is a good step to take.

For those who like to cook, trying out new WFPB recipes gradually and incorporating them into their routine is a great way to gradually make the change. For those who don't have the time or inclination to cook, frozen prepared vegan meals, veggie burgers, and other easy-to-prepare meal choices are a good start, as are the many different plant-based options available in many restaurants, especially in Mexican or Thai ones.

To help family members adopt this diet, she recommends,

> Food choices are extremely personal decisions. We want to feed ourselves and our families the diet that is best for their health, but at the same time, pushing new foods onto family members who are not ready to change the foods they eat can backfire. In my opinion, the best way to make the change is to explain to family members why you want or need to change your own diet first. And to set a good example by preparing plenty of healthy foods that you want to eat.
>
> If family members see a big improvement in your health because of changing your diet, that can be very motivating. In some family situations, telling family members who expect you to prepare their meals that they now must prepare their own meals if they want something different can also be an excellent motivator to accept the change in diet. Involving children in the cooking and giving them choices (all of which fit with a WFPB diet) can help give them a sense of control.
>
> Watching relevant documentaries together may inspire some family members and may help to counter many of the myths that persist in society about the need for meat protein. Hearing the facts from a source other than "Mom and Dad" can help, as can learning about other benefits of eating this way, such as for the animals and the environment.
>
> Ultimately, it's important to give family members control over their own diets so that they can proceed with changing their diet at their own pace and not feel pressured, even if that means that you have to eat and maybe prepare different foods from others in your family. Hopefully, you can still enjoy meals together and allow others to try your food if they express interest.

As society becomes more accepting of avoiding animal products, as more vegan products become available in stores and restaurants, as teenagers find that it's cool to be vegan, and as peer pressure to conform to traditional eating habits diminishes, this transition will become easier for everyone.[3]

Meet Gigi Carter

Carter has been WFPB since 2012. When asked what caused her to make the change to WFPB, she explains,

> My health journey started in 2007 when I was diagnosed with high cholesterol during a routine wellness exam. After a lipid panel and carotid artery scan, I was told that I had the arteries of a 46-year-old, but I was only thirty-five.
>
> I learned about the work of Dr. Dean Ornish and his Lifestyle Heart Trial, but my limiting beliefs at that time prevented me from giving up eating animal foods completely. Instead, over a five-year period (from 2007–2012), I followed what the government said was a healthy diet, opting for fish and poultry instead of beef. I switched to a low-fat dairy [diet] and was pretty good about consuming five servings of vegetables and fruits a day. While my cholesterol went from horrible to borderline bad, I never really fixed the problem. In addition, I was slowly putting on weight, and my energy level deteriorated.
>
> There were a few aha moments for me. The first one happened in 2011. My friend told me about the lemonade diet, or master cleanse, where you drink a concoction of lemon juice, cayenne pepper, and maple syrup for ten days. I did it about three times and lasted only five days.
>
> The protocol for coming off the master cleanse is to consume vegetable broth, raw veggies, and fruit for a few days before returning to your so-called healthy diet. What I noticed was that I felt best following the transition protocol of veggies and fruit. Not the master cleanse, not my regular diet, but those two to three days of just eating vegetable broth, raw veggies, and fruit.
>
> When my husband and I returned from a trip in January 2012, I made a public declaration that I was going vegetarian because, at this point, I thought I could give up meat but couldn't live without cheese. By June 2012, I did it!

> My lacto-ovo-vegetarian status lasted about a month. One weekend in July 2012, I watched two documentaries back-to-back: Forks Over Knives and Earthlings. Remembering what I learned about Dr. Ornish's Lifestyle Heart Trial years ago, the switch happened. I walked into the kitchen and told my husband, Kevin, that I was adopting a whole-food, plant-based vegan diet. To my delight and surprise, he said he'd do it with me.
>
> I made the change for two reasons:
>
> (1) I always claimed to be an animal lover, having rescued three dogs and supporting animal causes both with money and my volunteer time.
>
> (2) It was the right thing to do for my overall health.

When asked if she was vegan or WFPB, Carter states: "I consider myself a 'whole-food, plant-based vegan.' I eat healthy whole-plant foods and avoid processed vegan junk food. I choose vegan shoes, clothes, beauty products, and other items."

Carter finds that

> The people who have a strong 'why,' or the people who naturally march to the beat of their own drum are most successful at making this change. Peer and societal pressures to eat the Standard American Diet (SAD) are so strong that you must be grounded in your why for making the change or naturally just not care what other people think.
>
> Between overcoming food addictions and navigating family, friends, and coworkers who feel the need to control what you eat, it can be difficult to make the transition. But when you internalize the fact that it's not that you can't have this or that animal product but that you are choosing not to put that in your body, the feelings of deprivation are gone. That mindset shift is very powerful and life-changing.

She also says, "following a WFPB nutrition plan has made all the difference in my life, well beyond just lowering my cholesterol." Carter adds,

> [Specifically,] I'm postmenopausal and not on any prescription medications. I'm still racing bicycles and in the best shape of my life. Changing my diet

changed my life. It's also been an honor to be a part of my clients' health journeys. The weight loss, reversal of type 2 diabetes, lower cholesterol, reversal of hypertension, and improved mental and spiritual clarity are rewarding. My husband is doing very well with maintaining a healthy weight and being active with a WFPB lifestyle.

If you're on the fence about adopting a WFPB lifestyle, don't be. Just start with your next meal and immerse yourself in resources (books, podcasts, etc.) on the topic and seek support in the community. You'll soon find that you're gaining momentum toward a long-term healthy lifestyle.[4]

The evidence continues to prove that a WFPB diet is the healthiest way to eat to prevent and reverse chronic diseases and to help you age well. Hopefully, you now see how important your nutritional life is to your ability to be healthy and thrive.

Next, we'll move on to a discussion about our physical life.

CHAPTER 7

Your Physical Life

Exercise doesn't just slow the aging process; it can reverse it. Exercise is also medicine.

You can't be healthy without being physically active. If you are over forty years of age and aren't exercising on a regular basis, then it is time to make exercise a priority in your life and do it. If you have a chronic disease or other health issues, check with your doctor first.

"It's now considered 'normal' for people in their sixties and even seventies to run marathons," according to the Sherzais. Our expectations about aging have greatly changed in the last twenty years. We shouldn't accept an "outdated expectation of normal aging."[1] Don't accept inactivity and physical decline.

One study discovered that adults who participated in high physical activities had "a biologic aging advantage of nine years when compared to those who were sedentary, and seven years compared to those who were moderately active,"[2] explains Ornish. Highly active was described as 30–40 minutes of jogging a day, five days a week. Exercise has an "antiaging effect at a molecular level."

There are so many health reasons to exercise.

Physical exercise is more effective for increasing cognitive function than brain exercise, according to studies. Depression, anxiety, memory loss, dementia, diminished reaction time, and more can be stopped by physical exercise. The neurotransmitters freed during exercise develop brain function and slow the cognitive decline that happens in natural aging, advise Drs. Daniel Monti and Anthony Bazzan.[3]

Also, regular physical exercise can:

- Improve immune functioning so your body can resist disease
- Help you sleep better so you feel energized
- Reduce the risk of breast, prostate, and other cancers
- Decrease inflammation so you have less illness
- Keep your muscles and joints strong to help you stay injury-free and pain-free
- Promote good digestion and regularity
- Increase blood flow and vitality[4]

Daniel Monti, MD, MBA, is the founding director and the CEO of the Marcus Institute of Integrative Health, and Anthony Bazzan, MD, FACN, ABIHM, is the medical director of the Marcus Institute of Integrative Health.

Another study found that men and women with mild cognitive impairment (a precursor to Alzheimer's disease) who exercised four times a week for six months (treadmill, stationary bike, or elliptical machine) created more brain volume (measured by an MRI) and experienced an improvement in cognitive function, while the control group showed some brain atrophy and decreased cognitive function.[5]

Gotta Move More & Sit Less

Our bodies are built to move. Yet many of us are sedentary creatures with little or no real exercise in our lives. In fact, sitting is now called the new smoking, as it relates to health risks.[6] Today, many people sit for 13–15 hours a day, according to Andrew Jagim, PhD, a sports medicine professional and researcher.[7]

As a result of our sedentary lifestyle, we increase our risk of cancer, depression, lower cognitive ability, prediabetic blood sugar levels, diminished sex life, and sleep disruption, according to Lipman.[8]

Jagim suggests some ways you can add movement throughout your day:

- Use a standing desk
- Set an alarm to stand and move at least once per hour
- Walk during a lunch break
- Walk during phone calls
- Park far from store entrances
- Use the stairs, not the elevator
- Walk when doing routine tasks in your house, like brushing your teeth
- Walk your dog
- While watching TV, use a treadmill
- Perform work around the yard, plant a garden, and mow the grass[9]

The important thing is to move a lot throughout your day.

Exercise Lengthens Telomeres and Your Life

As telomeres shorten, so does your life. So it pays to get into the exercise habit.

"People who have consistently high levels of high physical activity have significantly longer telomeres than those who have sedentary lifestyles, and even longer than those who are moderately active,"[10] states Ornish.

In short, aerobic exercise is important for the entire body. "Many studies have shown that regular aerobic activity (defined as roughly 150 minutes per week of a moderate-intensity activity, like brisk walking) significantly reduces the risk of cardiovascular disease, type 2 diabetes, high blood pressure & high cholesterol, anxiety & depression, and obesity, all risk factors for cognitive decline,"[11] contend the Sherzais.

Also, chronic stress can greatly shorten telomeres, and exercise can reduce this risk. A study found that "postmenopausal women who exercised for at least 60 minutes, three or more times per week for about a year and a half had significantly longer telomeres than their sedentary peers. It showed the positive effects of both aerobic and resistance exercise,"[12] says Ornish.

Isn't it time that you started focusing on ways to lengthen your telomeres?

What Constitutes Aerobic Exercise?

Some aerobic activities you might want to consider:

- Take a brisk walk
- Mow the lawn or rake the leaves
- Learn to dance
- Walk to the store
- Hike a trail
- Do active forms of yoga
- Ride a bike (stationary or outdoors)
- Join a water aerobics class[13]

Strength Training Is Important as We Age

We don't want to lose muscle as we age, so muscle-strengthening activities are recommended two days a week. Some you might want to consider:

- Lifting weights
- Working with resistance bands
- Doing exercises using body weight for resistance (push-ups, sit-ups)
- Heavy gardening (digging, shoveling)
- Some types of yoga[14]

Get help from professionals to show you the correct way to do these activities and to make sure you aren't doing something that will hurt you. Should you inadvertently injure yourself, you can seek out osteopathic and orthopedic doctors who specialize in sports medicine and can advise you on rehab and recovery options, which can range from surgery to physical therapy. Using the correct form, starting with light weights, and increasing them as you build strength (but still maintaining form) will help you get the strength training benefits while maintaining a low risk of injury.

How Much and How Long?

According to the CDC website, adults 18–64 years need:

- For aerobic exercise—At least 150 minutes a week (for example, 30 minutes a day, 5 days a week of moderate-intensity activity, such as brisk walking). Or they need 75 minutes a week of vigorous-intensity activity, such as hiking, jogging, or running.
- For strength training—At least 2 days a week of activities that strengthen muscles.[15]

Adults sixty-five and older need the same as above except for the addition of activities to improve balance about three days a week.[16]

Aerobic activity gets you breathing harder and your heart beating faster. Depending on your health and fitness level, the key is to participate in a mild or vigorous intense activity. You might want to have a discussion with your doctor.

What is the Difference Between Moderate and Vigorous Aerobic Activity?

Considering a ten-point scale, zero is sitting, and ten is working as hard as you can; moderate would be a five. You can talk while doing performing the exercise but not sing a song. This is called the Talk Test.[17]

You don't have to do different types of exercise to prevent or turn around different diseases. Just find an activity that you enjoy. And DO IT! The more you move, the better you will feel and the more you will want to try other activities. And just ten minutes of exercise a week can make you happier. However, those that exercised (aerobic and stretching/balancing) thirty minutes a day showed the most benefit in increasing their happiness, contends Ornish.[18]

The Benefits of Simple Walking

Try to walk every day. While a gym provides a lot of benefits and options, nothing replaces getting outside, communing with nature. In addition to the physical aspects, there are also a lot of other benefits.

You would be amazed by the number of people who you will see: rain, shine, or snow. One such person is Janis Tremaine.

Janis Tremaine has been walking for thirty-two years! Previously, she participated in a pilates class two times a week, and that lasted for ten years. Then she decided she wanted to make a change. Janis wanted to exercise outside and whenever her schedule allowed.

"I walk for exercise. I think my mind and body need to work off stress. It's kind of a reset button. Walking helps clear my head. It's the best way to get the tension out of my shoulders. It's a great stress release and just gives me peace," reports Tremaine.

Her goal every day is to get her 10,000 steps in. She walks three miles in the morning and then the remaining 2,000 steps in either the mid-afternoon or after dinner.

When asked for any advice she would give to someone wanting to start, she offered, "I think the easiest way to begin an exercise plan is to walk. You can go with a friend or alone. You can spend as much time as you want. You don't need any special equipment, and you can go whenever it works with your schedule."[19] And that is all true! And a great reason to start walking!

Are you ready to lace up your exercise shoes and hit the streets or somewhere interesting?

Ready to Run a Marathon?

While still in her medical residency, Dr. Saray Stancic was diagnosed with multiple sclerosis (MS) at age twenty-eight. By her early thirties, she was dependent on a dozen medications (with horrible side effects), a cane, a walker, and crutches. She knew her future also included a wheelchair as the disease progressed, shares Dr. Stancic in her book *What's Missing from Medicine*.

One day, on the cover of a medical journal, she saw a picture of blueberries and the words "multiple sclerosis," and this prompted her research into a possible connection between diet and disease.

Next, she found a study by Dr. Roy Swank. In 1990, Swank reported that he had been treating MS patients with a low-fat, plant-based diet for over thirty years. The study found that his patients lived longer and better, with 95 percent remaining mobile and physically active. These were patients with MS, whom the medical community had given up on and labeled as progressive, debilitative, and incurable.

Stancic then researched the literature about MS. She knew genes played a big part in who got it. But she also understood (from medical school) the science of epigenetics and how the gene argument challenged that. Simply put, this means that just because you have a genetic predisposition to an illness doesn't necessarily mean that it will be expressed.

She started to investigate what turns the switch for MS and other chronic diseases. She discovered that diet, exercise, and stress activate certain genes. In short, the daily choices we make result in healthy outcomes or not.

With that knowledge, Stancic put together a plan to improve her diet by decreasing animal sources and processed food intake and eating healthier foods.

Next, she began an exercise plan she could do at home, practiced meditation to reduce stress, and learned ways to sleep without medications.

And with her commitment to her plan, Stancic started to improve and could reduce her medications. Her brother suggested she should think about running a marathon, so she started to learn to run, again. Even though she kept falling because her balance was off, she would continue to run at a nature preserve near her home.

Finally, on May 2, 2010, she crossed the finish line of the New Jersey Marathon. "It was one of the most joyful days of my life—not because it had been any kind of a lifelong goal to run a marathon but because I accomplished what seemed impossible just a few years earlier. My optimized lifestyle had been the critical key to my recovery, and implementing these modifications has changed the trajectory of my life."[20]

Carter Incorporates Exercise into Her Healthy Lifestyle

You met Gigi Carter in previous chapters. While in graduate school studying nutrition, she became a certified personal trainer because of the huge impact exercising was having on her health.

For Carter,

> *Exercise is a great stress reliever and helps me clear my head. I love the way it makes me feel, especially afterward. Exercise, along with diet, sleep, prayer/meditation, and love/support are vitally important for good health, a high quality of life, and longevity.*
>
> *Being consistent with exercise started after I changed what was on the end of my fork. Adopting a whole-food, plant-based vegan diet gave me the energy and pick-me-up that I never had throughout most of my adult life. I had so much energy, I started cycling and racing and continue to do so into my fifties.*
>
> *When I made the decision to dedicate the rest of my life to helping other women and a few good men take control of their health, I felt that included*

growing my skills to include both nutrition and physical activity. While I was starting the process to earn a master's in nutrition sciences from the University of Alabama at Birmingham, I also enrolled in courses and sat for the exam to become a certified personal trainer. Having this credential has helped me work with my nutrition clients to take their goals of healthy living to the next level.

When asked about the saying, "You can't out-exercise a bad diet," Carter states,

So very true! Many people struggle to give up the foods that are making them fat and sick because they don't want to admit they're addicted. They find comfort in those foods, even though those foods aren't solving their problems, feelings of loneliness, or boredom. They think that if they exercise more, it'll make up for poor dietary choices. Sadly, they go too long avoiding the root cause of their weight gain and illness. I know because I've been there. I've seen my clients struggle with this as well.[21]

Exercise is one of the pieces to a healthy life and not the only path (as many people think).

Start slowly and consult your doctor to ensure you are on a good regimen appropriate for you. Start where you are. If you need to start exercising ten minutes a day and work up to the CDC recommendation of thirty minutes, five days a week, then do that.[22] Now is the time to start to move and make it a habit! If you've been inactive, start small and go easy.

But start!

So what's your plan to incorporate aerobic exercise on a regular basis?

This concludes Chapter 7. Next, we'll discuss the importance environment has on your health.

CHAPTER 8
Environment Matters

Do You Live in a Soul-Nourishing Space?

Have you recognized that your home impacts your quality of life? How do you feel in your home? Alive, energized, at peace, or depleted, depressed, and confused? A chaotic house equals a chaotic mind.

Self-care includes taking the time and the resources to create a home that feeds your soul: beautiful (however that feels to you), tidy, organized, and—most of all—clean.

According to Cheryl Richardson, creating a soul-nourishing environment can literally transform a person's life.[1] Richardson authored *The Art of Extreme Self-Care*.

So, how and where do you start to create this soul-nourishing life? You can start by analyzing those thing in your home that you love or need and getting rid of the rest. While you can find specialty books written describing intricate ways to declutter your house, it doesn't need to be complicated. Just ask yourself, do you love it or need it? If not, get rid of it and let it serve someone else. Stacks of things have no place in a soul-nourishing home. Go through all your stuff (with nothing off-limits) and get rid of what you don't love or need. And make it a rule *not* to save anything simply because you might need it in the future. Usually, you don't.

You may discover as you get farther on your journey that much of the stuff simply doesn't fit the person you have become or the person you want to be.

You may find that "less is more" when it comes to your surroundings. It's quite a change in perspective!

Don't forget to go through your files. Find out what papers you need to keep and get rid of the rest. Shred properly with a trusted company.

Richardson advises us to consider the following when thinking about the space we live in, going one room at a time, and write down the answers:

- *What do these surroundings say about you?*
- *Do they reflect the essence of who you are?*
- *If this space were to tell a story about your life, what story would it tell?*
- *How does this space make you feel?*
- *What have you been tolerating for too long?*
- *What areas make you feel good?*
- *What areas make you feel bad? Why?*
- *If you could sweep the whole room into the trash and start over, would you?*[2]

Now that you have the information you need, you can get to work.

Start with a clean canvas and spend time exploring to see what you want to create overall. And create a plan for each room to make sure all flows well. This can take some time and shouldn't be rushed. Make it a priority to create a space that "feels" right to you.

So, is your home a soul-nourishing space? Or is it time for a change?

Setting Your Environment Up for Success

An organized environment matters! If you want to make healthy lifestyle changes, your environment needs to be designed to support your healthy lifestyle aspirations. This will enable you to have a better chance of succeeding.

A Healthy Home. High self-esteem is important in deciding to create and maintain a healthy home. You need to believe that you deserve a healthy environment to go with your healthy lifestyle.

A healthier home is clean, clutter-free, and organized. It is amazing how much better we feel once we have eliminated "the stuff" in our lives to make room for healthier options. Once everything is organized and clean, it is so much easier to keep it that way.

Kitchen. It's important to have the right food in your home to support your healthy lifestyle from the beginning. To be able to eat healthy, make sure you have emptied all the unhealthy food from your environment. It is so easy to go back to junk food. Research is showing that our brains are wired for junk food and the sugar in it. [3]

Exercise Clothing. A great tip is to have your exercise clothes organized so grabbing them in the morning (or whatever time you go) is easy and requires no big choices or actions looking for things. Consider keeping your gym clothes (and pre-packed bag) in one designated spot and walking clothes in another. If you know you need to get it done, make it easy for yourself to do so!

Support from Others. If you live with others, it is important to enlist their support. Hopefully, they will participate in the adventure with you and become healthier in the process. Unfortunately, it can be an uphill battle if they aren't supportive. You can also find an accountability partner. You would be amazed how that little action can keep you committed to your lifestyle changes.

Minimize Exposure to Toxins

It is difficult to have a healthy life without minimizing your exposure to hazardous toxins in your home and everyday beauty products.

Neal Barnard, MD, FACC, author of *Your Body in Balance: The New Science of Food, Hormones, and Health*, says it is also important to avoid environmental chemicals and become aware of toxic chemicals we encounter in everyday life:

- **BPA**—*found in resins that line food cans and hard, clear plastics and thermal papers (receipts printed at cash registers, gas pumps, dry cleaners, etc.)*
- **Phthalates**—*used to make plastics bend. Phthalates dissolve in food containers, especially in fatty foods like milk, butter, meat, and cheese.*
- **Pesticides**—*Monsanto's Roundup, active ingredient glyphosate, is the most popular weed killer. Also, atrazine (the second leading herbicide) is used as a weed killer for corn and sorghum used in animal feed and is sprayed on lawns and golf courses.*
- **PCBs**—*synthetic chemicals banned in the US in 1977. Still present in the environment and can be found in dairy products, meat, and eggs.*
- **Citric acid**—*a chemical additive used by food manufacturers. Nearly all are made in Chinese factories using a fermentation process with mold, and mold ends up in the end product and can trigger allergic or autoimmune reactions. Can be seen frequently on food and beverage labels, or even in toothpaste.*
- **Pesticides and industrial chemicals found in rivers and oceans**—*Fish ingest these chemicals, and they accumulate in their body fat. "A study of 431 overweight women and men found that those with the highest levels of chemical pollutants in their bloodstreams were most likely to have elements of metabolic syndrome—the combination of problems with body weight, blood pressure, blood sugar, and blood lipids" according to Barnard.*
- **Hormones in meat and dairy production**—*In the US and other countries, hormones (testosterone, estradiol, progesterone, and three synthetic hormones—zeranol, melengestrol acetate, and trenbolone acetate) are routinely used in meat and dairy production. Also, in the US, some dairy farmers inject their cows with a genetically engineered bovine growth hormone (bovine somatotropin) to increase milk production.*[4]

Ways to Avoid Environmental Chemicals in Your Food

Barnard also advises that we select organic produce to minimize exposure to toxins. Because of the pesticide residue on conventionally grown produce, the Environmental Working Group (EWG.org) publishes a list of the fruits and vegetables we need to purchase organic:

- Strawberries
- Spinach
- Kale
- Nectarines
- Apples
- Grapes
- Peaches
- Cherries
- Pears
- Tomatoes
- Celery
- Potatoes
- Hot Peppers

The list above does change, so you should check the website EWG.org for updated information. And you can get the list of the Clean 15 for when it isn't as important to purchase organic. Also, organic produce, by law, cannot be genetically modified. [5]

Additional Protection Against Environmental Chemicals

We can't avoid all exposures to chemicals in today's world due to their extensive use in agriculture, industry, and commercial manufacturing. However, Barnard recommends there are some protections we can take to minimize them. And the best way to protect yourself from environmental chemicals is to start with a healthy plant-based diet. Additional suggestions include:

- *Don't consume animal products. Environmental chemicals can be found in animal tissues.*
- *Choose organic produce, especially those labeled as the Dirty Dozen on the Environmental Working Group's website (EWG.org).*

- *Use canned products labeled "BPA-free" and choose fresh or frozen products instead of canned.*
- *Use glass not plastic in the microwave.*
- *Use only BPA-free designated plastics. A number 3 or 7 on the product means that it may contain BPA unless it is labelled BPA-free.*
- *Drink the cleanest water you can. Spring water is better than tap. And if you use a tap, filters can remove pollutants. Effective filters should have an NSF certification marking indicating that the product meets the American National Standards Institute's Standard 53 for the reduction of volatile organic compounds, including atrazine and other pollutants.*
- *Don't handle thermal receipts if you don't need them. Many people don't know that they contain BPA. Wear gloves if you do handle them.*
- *Read labels on all personal care products. Try to use those with the minimum number of additives.*[6]

Toxic Ingredients in Skin Care Products

Though not an exhaustive list, here are some of the toxic ingredients in skin care products to keep out of your life, according to Deepak Chopra and Kimberly Synder:

- Benzoyl peroxide
- Synthetic (or artificial) FD&C colors & dyes
- Propylene glycol (PG) & butylene glycol
- Diethanolamine (DEA), monoethanolamine (MEA), & triethanolamine (TEA)
- Methyl, butyl, ethyl, & propyl parabens
- Sodium lauryl sulfate (SLS) & sodium laureth sulfate (SLES)
- Dioxin
- Polyethylene glycol (PEG)
- Avobenzone
- Phthalates
- Triclosan

- DMDM hydantoin & imidazolidinyl urea[7]

For more information, visit the websites for the campaign for Safe Cosmetics (safecosmetics.org) and the Environmental Working Group Skin Deep Cosmetics Database (ewg.org/skindeep). These organizations believe that toxic ingredients:

- Can cause DNA damage
- Act as carcinogens
- Create brain, liver, kidney, and other organ abnormalities
- Produce allergic or other reactions
- Cause eye damage, nervous system damage, reproductive damage, and birth defects

What changes are you going to make to improve your environment?

Your Virtual World

Technology has undoubtedly fulfilled the promise of making our lives easier. You can literally accomplish in minutes things that used to take hours or days. You have a world of information at your fingertips. You can read about any subject without spending hours researching in a library. You can learn how to do almost anything by watching videos. Pay bills in seconds (or set up auto-pay) instead of writing checks, addressing envelopes, and licking stamps. Have almost anything you want delivered to your doorstep in a day or two. Watch movies, keep in touch with friends on the other side of the planet, set up an entire travel itinerary from your recliner. These truly are amazing times in which we live!

But there's a dark side to all this convenience. Technology saves us so much time and effort, but what are you doing with all those savings? For many people, it's continued engagement with the virtual world, which provides little benefit compared to the real world. In fact, it's becoming increasingly clear that it not only provides little benefit but is also capable of causing significant damage.

On an individual level, social media use has been associated with an increase in depression and anxiety. On a broader social scale, it has resulted in deep societal rifts that are fed by algorithms designed to keep us engaged but produce echo-chamber environments where people are increasingly comfortable entrenching themselves in their opinions, vilifying all who disagree with them and reducing public discourse to memes and hashtags reflecting half-truths and sometimes out-and-out lies. There seems to be little desire to pursue truth or recognize that problems are complex and nuanced.

All of this is to say that, in addition to paying close attention to what you consume in your physical diet, you need to pay close attention to what you consume in your mental diet.

- Take inventory of the time you spend in the "virtual world." Watching a few videos here and there and scrolling through your Facebook feed often takes up way more time than you realize. Ask yourself if that time could be better spent. Would it be more beneficial to take a walk or meet a friend for coffee?

- Consider reducing your time spent on social media. Do a "social media detox" where you disengage from social media for thirty days and see how that feels when you're done.

- Pay close attention to your sources of news. Are they reliable? The barrier for publishing anything on the internet is extremely low. Journalistic integrity is a thing of the past, so don't assume that what you're reading is true. Is your news biased?[8] What is the other side saying? Use critical thinking and question what you're reading instead of accepting it on blind faith.

- Actively seek out opinions and perspectives that differ from your own. While you may not be influenced to change your opinion, perhaps it will at least provide you with some understanding about how differing opinions arise. This can help raise the level of discourse. You don't have to agree with the other side, but it helps if you can respect them.

- While this is not a book on cyber security, it's worth mentioning that you need to take extra precautions to keep your data and finances safe. There are many bad actors out there looking for opportunities to scam you out of your money. Ensure that you keep your passwords private and protected and treat all email correspondence with skepticism. Never click on links in emails but instead go directly to websites to do your business. Likewise, never give out credit card information on the phone unless *you* initiated the call and you know who you're dealing with.

What changes need to be made in your environment to support your healthy lifestyle aspirations?

CHAPTER 9

Beauty Redefined

The definition of beauty changes as we age, so here are some ways to think about it differently.

Things like fashion and beauty may be important for many women. Aging gracefully doesn't mean that you no longer care about how you look, but you also have to embrace aging and beauty in a different way. Many women can struggle with this.

The secret is that . . . it's an inside job. It isn't about external validation. Instead, beauty is internal self-confidence.

A Different Way to Think About Beauty

Dr. Sherrie Campbell's wise words:

> There is no doubt that there is great value to external beauty. For some, how they look physically is simply an expression and celebration of their internal beauty, but often those who are physically attractive are emotionally unattractive. To be beautiful inside and out, you must possess more than a pretty shell.
>
> Here are ten understated qualities of beauty:
>
> - **Elegance:** Elegance is that dignified grace about your appearance, movement, personal style, or behavior. To be elegant is to be strong and assured in who you are and to move gently within that energy.

- **Kindness:** The kindness of your spirit; how you treat, think about, and speak to others from a genuine and sensitive place. You are kind, even to those whom you do not care for. You are aware that you can love someone even if you do not like them.

    Being kind may be perceived as a weakness or vulnerability by others, but you know that kindness is one of your strongest influences. If you can't say something nice, you have control to remain quiet.

- **Composure:** Composure is the beauty of self-control. Life is always going to bring its challenges. Without a sense of composure, it is easy to allow conflict situations and relationships to unnerve you, but when you have composure, you understand the concept of less equals more.

    The less you react, defend, explain, or become fearful or controlling, the more command you have over a situation. Having composure allows you to stand tall with grace in the face of loss and challenges and not be overly boastful when it comes to success.

- **Courage:** Be willing to dare greatly in your life. It takes courage to love fully, to change yourself when necessary, to feel deeply, to leave love when it's scary, and to chase your dreams with passion and unwavering tenacity.

- **Confident:** When you are self-loving, you naturally possess a quiet confidence. Your self-awareness, dedication to self-development, and personal growth provide you the knowledge to succeed at nearly anything you seek.

- **Deliberate:** You are clear and persistent about who you are, where you are headed in life, and what you want from your relationships to be happy. In being deliberate, people know where they stand with you. You get what you want in life because you are clear in saying what you want.

    You use each challenge life brings to positively refine yourself. This refinement keeps your life clean of negativity. Being deliberate keeps you pointed in the direction of your dreams, connected to your true loves, and living genuinely as who you are.

    In being deliberate, your life is not set up on pretenses. Who you are does not change from person to person or situation to situation.

- **Intelligent:** Intelligence is about knowledge, but even more so about emotions. In being aware of your emotional patterns, you are endowed with the flexibility to handle challenges and changes, allowing you to unlock smart solutions to your problems.

- **Humble:** Life isn't all about you; in fact, you prefer to celebrate the accomplishments of others as much as your own. You are proud of who you are but have no need to add histrionics to your success. Most of the time, you prefer being in the background, working hard, and allowing your success to speak for itself.

  You are sensitive and want the best for everyone. You do not see yourself above others, as you are secure enough in yourself that the trap of comparison doesn't interest you. You enjoy your life for what it is and do not feel entitled to more without the commensurate work to back it up.

- **Honest:** People gravitate toward what is real. You are simple, up-front, [and] gentle, but direct in the 'being' of who you are. You are content to live life patiently and know how to wait well. For you, life is about being authentic and following your heart and nothing else.

  You are someone others can depend upon, as you have no ulterior motives. You are relationship-oriented, not agenda-oriented. You believe the truth is the only path to success and deep intimacy.

- **Loving:** There is nothing more appealing to others than to be in the presence of a loving person. When you love yourself, you have endless love to give. For you, love is a verb, and it expresses itself through loving kindness, touch, your smile, and a sense of inner joy and vitality.

  You are warm toward others and kind to yourself. There is nothing you wouldn't do to help, and this loving approach is taken into every area of your life from career to parenting. Further, you apply love as a form of discipline and set boundaries when necessary. There are times when the only way another can learn and grow is for you either to withdraw your love or to set boundaries around it, to protect your generous nature.

  Love is not just a gentle emotion; it is also firm. You know that for you to remain loving, you must protect your heart and put yourself first in negative *situations. Through life's experiences, you have come to learn that some people can stay in your heart, but not in your life.*

To be truly beautiful [as you age], it is these understated qualities of beauty, which are sustaining. To possess any of these will increase your beauty exponentially [as you age]. Who you are internally is the marker of your impact on the world. Let the kindness of your character say more about you than what you see in the mirror.[1]

Next, it is time to create your customized plan to take charge of your health and aging.

CHAPTER 10
Conclusion

Time to Create Your Customized Plan

In this book, we have shared with you the many ways that you can change your life to become much healthier tomorrow than you are today. We have shared numerous ideas and resources throughout the book that you can use as a guide to healthy aging. We hope we have stirred your curiosity so that you will follow up to learn more from them. Honestly, they are nuggets of gold.

This book is our presentation of a new path to aging with words that include thriving instead of declining. We can't stop aging, but we can control *how* we age as it relates to our health.

We have tried to create a healthy aging beginner's manual for you. And as with most manuals, we hope it is one you keep coming back to as you progress on your journey and are ready to take on new challenges.

It can take years to make the changes that we have shared. It is an iterative process; the better you feel, the healthier you become, the more changes you are inclined to make. So keep with it and don't get discouraged by roadblocks and backslides.

Now is your time to take the next step to action. What would you like to try?

Remember to start small and realize it is a journey, not a destination. Also, keep in mind:

- The food you eat is the foundation for a healthy life.
- Give everything two months before you move on to try something new.
- Find an accountability partner or coach to keep you on track.
- Create S.M.A.R.T. goals (specific, measurable, attainable, realistic, and timely) around the changes you want to make.
- Be kind to yourself. It is okay to fail and start again. Think of the failures as lessons learned. And start again. Get help if you need it.
- You don't have to feel motivated to get started. Just begin.
- And always, especially if you have serious health issues, make the changes in partnership with your PCP.

Finally, don't forget, your health is real wealth. With the limited years that you have left on this earth, how do you want to spend your time? Managing chronic disease or terminal illness or living the longest life with the fewest years of disability?

Your Customized Plan

Define what healthy means for you. And why is this important?

What is your passion or purpose that can serve as your North Star to keep you on track? Write it down and put it where you can see it every day.

Document where you are now from Chapter 1:

- Known risk factors?
- Any chronic diseases or health issues that you have?
- Current biometric readings: height, weight, body mass index (BMI), blood pressure, blood cholesterol, and blood sugar?

What specific changes would you like to happen in reference to the above question?

Go Back and Review the Chapters

- What must you do to ensure you have a health-care team in place?
- What is the first change you want to make in your emotional/mental life?
- What is the first change you want to make in your nutritional life?
- What is the first change you want to make in your physical life?
- What is the first change you want to make in your environment?

There is your customized plan. But for real change to occur, *you have to take action.*

We thank you for reading our book. Please help us make the world a healthier place! If you know someone who could benefit from this information, please gift them a book or tell them about it. And if you want to connect with us more, please visit our businesses:

Debbye Omlie
www.debbyeomlie.com
Debbye is passionate about helping people live healthy lifestyles.

Blake Anderson
www.HonuPerspective.com
Blake utilizes neuro-transformational coaching techniques to help his clients achieve their goals through lasting lifestyle changes.

Finally, we wish you blessings and good health as you take steps to control your health to prevent or reverse chronic disease in your life and age well, thriving!

For more information (aside from that listed throughout the book) or to find allies or a support group to help you, check out the Resources section.

DISCLAIMER: Please be aware that this book's materials and content are for general information only and are not intended to be a substitute for professional medical advice, diagnosis, or treatment. Readers of this book should not rely on the information provided for their own health needs. All specific questions should be presented to your healthcare provider(s).

Resources

We highly recommend the resources below that we have found most helpful.

Forks Over Knives Website

www.forksoverknives.com

Forks Over Knives became a spark for national change. The film was a hit. The accompanying book became a *New York Times* No. 1 bestseller.

Recipes, articles, health topics, meal planners, cooking courses, and a beginner's guide are on the website. You can also stream the *Forks Over Knives* documentary for free.

Healthy World Vitality Plan

http://hwvitality.com

"Small Group Support for Healthy Vital Lives"

This plan is sponsored by Healthy World Sedona. It creates small groups that educate and support individuals so they can make and sustain the kind of lifestyle changes that enable people to live their healthiest, most vital lives.

You can enroll in a ten-week small support group online (can live anywhere) for a nominal fee. The fee includes a trained nutritional coach, information, and assessment tools across the lifestyle realms of nutrition, exercise, stress management, restorative sleep, and optimal cognitive activity. Group members can then determine the steps they need to take to prevent, improve, or even eliminate chronic conditions and restore health.

Live *Lunch and Learn* sessions with nationally known speakers, as well as cooking tips and demos, are also included. A resource section on the website lists books, cookbooks, movies, videos, and personalized cooking classes and coaching for more information and help about the WFPB diet and lifestyle.

Modern Elder Academy (MEA)

www.modernelderacademy.com

If you need help determining your purpose or answering the "what's next" question, you'll find help at MEA.

MEA is on a mission to build a community of inspired and empowered midlifers and reframe midlife from a crisis to a calling. It is the world's first wisdom school. MEA provides an environment to reimagine midlife as a time for learning, growth, and positive transformation through immersive workshops and sabbaticals.

Nutrition Facts Website

www.nutritionfacts.org

This is a science-based nonprofit organization founded by Michael Greger, MD, MD, that provides free updates on the latest in nutrition research via bite-size podcasts, videos, blogs, and infographics. It is a non-commercial public service.

Physicians Committee for Responsible Medicine

www.pcrm.org

Great information covering nutrition, health topics and disease states, plant-based diets, ethical science, and research is on the website.

The ExamRoom podcast is another great place for information and can be found at www.pcrm.org/podcast.

PlantStrong

PlantStrong seeks to simplify the journey to a whole-food, plant-based lifestyle with a complete ecosystem of education, support, and delicious meal solutions.

The *Plant-Strong* podcast with Rip Esselstyn is also informative and can be found at www.plantstrongpodcast.com.

Featured in the Book:

Chris Kalinich

Kalinich is a certified functional nutritionist and culinary nutrition educator at sedonatruenutrition.com. She is a member of the National Association of Nutrition Professionals and the American College of Lifestyle Medicine.

Amanda Strombom

Strombom is the president of *Vegetarians of Washington*. She has written or co-authored over 37 research review articles, which have been published in medical journals, on a special website—pbdmedicine.org—and in a book for physicians.

Gigi Carter

Carter is the co-founder of *Healthy for My Purpose*, a wellness practice that helps faith-minded women use the Daniel Fast as a jumping-off point for a healthy, long-term, plant-based lifestyle. Carter is a licensed nutritionist in the state of Washington, a fitness specialist, and a member of the American College of Lifestyle Medicine. She has a certificate in plant-based nutrition from Cornell University. She is also the author or co-author of the books, *The Plant-Based Workplace, Daniel Fast: Why You Should Only Do It Once,* and *The Spinach in My Teeth*.

Blake Anderson

Honu Perspective Life and Wellness Coaching

www.HonuPerspective.com

This is the Life and Wellness coaching practice of co-author Blake Anderson.

The acquisition of knowledge is only half the battle when it comes to improving your health. After reading this book, you should have an idea of what a healthier life looks like for you and what you need to do. The other half of the battle is making the changes *you now know you need to make* to support the life you want.

Honu Perspective is for you if you want to . . .

- Identify and face your fears, most likely the biggest things holding you back, and *overcome them*.
- Love and accept yourself, which is necessary for *experiencing breakthroughs*.
- Not only accept failure but anticipate it and embrace it as a *critical component of growth*.
- Eliminate limiting beliefs and *discover your full potential*.

- Establish foundational processes and habits that *produce lasting results.*
- Quiet the noise and shed the chaos that life throws your way to *create balance for yourself.*
- Envision a future for yourself and *overcome resistance to change.*
- Get yourself unstuck and *generate energy for forward movement.*

. . . with an experienced coach who is client-focused, practical, supportive, and provides a safe, judgment-free environment for you to grow and thrive.

Debbye Omlie

www.debbyeomlie.com

Debbye helps people live their longest, healthiest lives

Healthy Aging Adventures

The art of starting! Decide to draw a line in the sand and say, "No more. I am going to make changes in my life to be healthy." Are you strapped for time to learn how to be healthy, or have you had it with feeling tired and irritable with less joy in your life? Need some "me" time to figure it out?

Join this immersive experience to learn the critical healthy aging concepts on your journey to becoming healthy! This day and a half over a weekend will walk you through the topics using evidence-based information.

Omlie demystifies the healthy aging process and provides practical, evidence-based information to use in a fun, easy-to-learn environment and experience.

We will help you create the initial steps towards your path.

You will:

- Learn the main concepts of being and staying healthy
- Identify emotional/mental blocks standing in your way
- Start to identify your passion or purpose for living longer
- Taste whole food, plant-based foods
- Move your body
- Connect with like-minded people
- Create a mini-plan, next steps for after you leave
- Have fun!

More information is on the website.

Endnotes

Introduction

[1] Stephen Kopecky. *Live Longer Younger: 6 Steps to Prevent Heart Disease, Cancer, Alzheimer's, Diabetes, and More* (Rochester: Mayo Clinic Press, 2021), 25.

[2] the website for Cleveland Clinic; Health Essentials; "Five Healthy Habits that Prevent Chronic Disease"; 5 Healthy Habits That Prevent Chronic Disease – Cleveland Clinic , posted Sept. 2, 2020.

[3] the website for WorldHealth.net; "Bloomberg's Global Health Index for 2020;" https://worldhealth.net/news/bloombergs-global-health-index-2020/, posted June 18, 2020.

[4] the website for the Centers for Disease Control and Prevention; National Center for Health Statistics; "Percent of U.S. Adults 55 and Over with Chronic Conditions"; https://www.cdc.gov/nchs/health_policy/adult_chronic_conditions.htm ,last reviewed Nov. 6, 2015.

[5] the website for the Centers for Disease Control and Prevention; National Center for Health Statistics; "Percent of U.S. Adults 55 and Over with Chronic Conditions;" https://www.cdc.gov/nchs/health_policy/adult_chronic_conditions.htm, last reviewed Nov. 6, 2015.

[6] the website for TIME; Health. Heart Health; "Women Die from Heart Attacks More Often Than Man. Here's Why – And What Doctors Are Doing About it." https://time.com/5499872/women-heart-disease/ posted April 1, 2019.

[7] the website for T. Colin Campbell Center for Nutritional Studies; "COVID-19 and Code Blue, A Timely Intersection;" https:nutritionstudies.org/covid-19-and-code-blue-a-timely-intersection/ posted July 17, 2020, by Saray Stancic, July 17, 2020.

[8] T. Colin Campbell, PhD and Howard Jacobson, PhD, *Whole. Rethinking the Sciences of Nutrition* (Dallas: BenBella Books, Inc., 2013), 4.

Chapter 2

[1] the website for Harvard Medical School; Harvard Health Publishing; Harvard Health (blog); "Why Do You Need a Primary Care Physician?," https://www.health.harvard.edu/blog/why-do-you-need-a-primary-care-physician-2019081917527, by Peter Gonzalez, MD, posted Aug. 19, 2019.

[2] the website for National Institute on Aging; National Institutes of Health (NIH); " How to Choose a Doctor You Can Talk to;" https://www.nia.nih.gov/health/how-choose-doctor-you-can-talk, content reviewed Feb. 1, 2020.

[3] the website for the American Academy of Family Physicians; family doctor.org; "Choosing a Family Doctor," https://familydoctor.org/choosing-a-family-doctor/ created by family doctor.org editorial staff & reviewed by Deepak S. Patel, MD, FAAFP, FACSM.

[4] the website for National Institute on Aging; National Institutes of Health (NIH); " How to Choose a Doctor You Can Talk to, Choose a Doctor" https://www.nia.nih.gov/health/how-choose-doctor-you-can-talk#choose, content reviewed Feb. 1, 2020.

[5] the website for the American College of Lifestyle Medicine; "Definition of Lifestyle Medicine;" https://lifestylemedicine.org/overview/.

[6] the website for Global Wellness Institute; "What is Wellness? Wellness Continuum https://globalwellnessinstitute.org/what-is-wellness/.

[7] the website for Honu Perspective; FAQ page; "What is Wellness?" https://honuperspective.com/faq.

Chapter 3

[1] Brene' Brown, PhD, MSW, *The Gifts of Imperfection*.(Center City: Hazelden Publishing, 2010, 2020). 114.

[2] Kopecky, Live Longer Younger, 58.

[3] Kopecky, S. Live Longer Younger, iv-v.

[4] Bill Burnett and Dave Evans, *Designing Your Life How to Build a Well-Lived, Joyful Life* (New York: Alfred A. Knopf; 2016), xvi.

[5] Will Bulsiewicz, *Fiber Fueled. The Plant-Based Health Program for Losing Weight, Restoring Your Health, and Optimizing Your Microbiome* (New York: Avery, 2020), 173 -174.

[6] Carol Dweck, PhD, *Mindset-The New Psychology of Success* (New York: Ballantine Books,2016), 7.

[7] Dean Ornish, MD and Anne Ornish, *Undo It! How Simple Lifestyle Changes Can Reverse Most Chronic Diseases* (New York: Ballantine Books, 2019), 143.

[8] Ornish and Ornish, *Undo It!*, 143-145.

[9] the website for the Greater Good Science Center at UC Berkeley; "The Science of Gratitude;" A white paper prepared for the John Templeton Foundation, May 2018, https://ggsc.berkeley.edu/images/uploads/GGSC-JTF_White_Paper-Gratitude-FINAL.pdf by Summer Allen, PhD.

[10] the website for Harvard Medical School; Harvard Health Publishing; Harvard Health (blog); "Giving Thanks Can Make You Happier;" https://

www.health.harvard.edu/healthbeat/giving-thanks-can-make-you-happier.

[11] Kopecky, *Live Younger Longer*, 80-81.

[12] Bulsiewicz W. *Fiber Fueled*, 199.

[13] the website for TED, Ideas Worth Spreading; "The Three Secrets of Resilient People;" https://www.ted.com/talks/lucy_hone_the_three_secrets_of_resilient_people August 2019, Lucy Hone.

[14] the website for SleepFoundation.org; How Sleep Works; "Why Do We Need Sleep?;" https://www.sleepfoundation.org/articles/why-do-we-need-sleep, updated Dec. 8, 2023, by Danielle Pacheco and Dr. Abhinav Singh.

[15] the website for SleepFoundation.org; Physical Health and Sleep; "How Sleep Affects Immunity," https://www.sleepfoundation.org/articles/how-sleep-affects-your-immunity, updated Aug. 15, 2023, by Eric Suni and Dr. Kimberly Truong.

[16] Frank Lipman MD and Amely Greeven, *How to Be Well. The 6 Keys to a Happy and Healthy Life* (Boston: Houghton Mifflin Harcourt, 2018), 115.

[17] Lipman and Greeven, *How to Be Well*, 113.

[18] Lipman and Greeven, *How to Be Well*, 108-109.

[19] Dean Sherzai MD and Ayesha Sherzai MD, *The Alzheimer's Solution. A Breakthrough Program to Prevent and Reverse the Symptoms of Cognitive Decline at Every Age (*New York: Harper On, 2017), 7.

[20] Sherzai and Sherzai, The Alzheimer's Solution, 11.

[21] Sherzai and Sherzai, The Alzheimer's Solution, 242-243.

[22] Brene' Brown, *The Gifts of Imperfection, Letting Go of Who You Think You're Supposed to Be and Embrace Who You Are* (Center City: Hazelden Publishing, 2010), 100.

[23] Stuart Brown MD and Christopher Vaughan C, *Play. How It Shapes the Brain, Opens the Imagination, and Invigorates the Soul* (New York: Avery, 2009), 215.

[24] Brown and Vaughan, *Play,* 7.

[25] Brown and Vaughan, *Play,* 7-8.

[26] Brown and Vaughan, *Play,* 11.

[27] Brown and Vaughan, *Play.* 17.

[28] Burnett and Evans, *Designing a Life You Love,* 15.

[29] Burnett and Evans, *Designing a Life You Love.* 15.

[30] Ornish and Ornish, *Undo It!,* 196.

[31] Ornish and Ornish, *Undo It!,* 197.

Chapter 4

[1] Oprah Winfrey, *The Path Made* Clear. Your Life's Direction and Purpose (New York: Flatiron Books, 2019), 10.

[2] Michael Arloski, PhD, *Wellness Coaching for Lasting Lifestyle Change 2nd Ed.* (Duluth; Whole Person, 2014), 27.

[3] Kopecky, *Live Younger Longer,* 78.

[4] Lipman and Greeven, *How to Be Well,* 239.

[5] Kopecky, *Live Younger Longer,* 79.

[6] the website for The Guardian (US edition, Guardian Media Group); "A New Start After 60; I Trained to be a Flight Attendant – it's the Only Way I Could Explore the World" https://www.theguardian.com/lifeandstyle/2022/apr/25/a-

new-start-after-60-i-trained-to-be-a-flight-attendant-its-the-only-way-i-could-explore-the-world, April 25, 2022, by Paula Cocozza.

[7] the website for The Guardian (US edition, Guardian Media Group); "A New Start After 60; I Trained to be a Flight Attendant – it's the Only Way I Could Explore the World" https://www.theguardian.com/lifeandstyle/2022/apr/25/a-new-start-after-60-i-trained-to-be-a-flight-attendant-its-the-only-way-i-could-explore-the-world, April 25, 2022, by Paula Cocozza.

[8] Ornish and Ornish, *UnDo It!*, 237.

[9] the website for the World Health Organization; "A Global Strategy for Healthy Ageing," Kalache, Alexandre & Kickbusch, Ilona (1997); published in *World Health*, 50 (4), 4-5. World Health Organization, https://apps.who.int/iris/handle/10665/330616 .

Chapter 5

[1] Kopecky, *Live Younger Longer*, 95.

[2] Bulsiewicz, *Fiber-Fueled*, 12-13.

[3] Gigi Carter, *The Plant-Based Workplace. Add Profits, Engage Employees and Save the Planet* (Eastsound: Gigi Carter through Amazon Publishing, 2018), 54.

[4] Ornish and Ornish, *UnDo It!*, 62.

[5] T. Colin Campbell, PhD and Nelson Disla, *The Future of Nutrition* (Dallas: Benbella Books, 2020), p.7.

[6] Campbell and Disla, *The Future of Nutrition*, 7-9.

[7] Sherzai and Sherzai, *The Alzheimer's Solution*, 3.

[8] Sherzai and Sherzai, *The Alzheimer's Solution*, 2.

⁹ Sherzai and Sherzai, *The Alzheimer's Solution,* 81-82.

¹⁰ Sherzai and Sherzai, *The Alzheimer's Solution,* 57.

¹¹ the website for Harvard Medical School; Harvard Health Publishing; Harvard Health (blog); "Staying Healthy; Healthy Diet Associated with Lower COVID-19 Risk and Severity," https://www.health.harvard.edu/staying-healthy/harvard-study-healthy-diet-associated-with-lower-covid-19-risk-and-severity, by Heidi Godman, Dec. 1, 2021.

¹² Campbell and Jacobson, *Whole,* 198-199.

¹³ Campbell and Jacobson, *Whole,* 202-203.

Chapter 6

¹ Rod Horn, email message to author (Omlie), March 19, 2023.

² Chris Kalinich, email message to author (Omlie), July 5, 2022.

³ Amanda Strombom, email message to author (Omlie), July 12, 2022.

⁴ Gigi Carter, email message to author (Omlie), July 29, 2022.

Chapter 7

¹ Sherzai and Sherzai, *The Alzheimer's Solution,* 145.

² Ornish and Ornish, *UnDo It!,* 103.

³ Daniel Monti, MD and Anthony Bazzan, MD, *Tapestry of Health. Weaving Wellness into Your Life Through the New Science of Integrative Medicine (*San Diego: Kales Press, 2020), 99-100.

⁴ Monti and Bazzan, *Tapestry of Health,* 100.

[5] Ornish and Ornish, *UnDo It!*, 107.

[6] the website for the Better Health Channel, "The Dangers of Sitting: Why Sitting is the New Smoking"; https://www.betterhealth.vic.gov.au/health/healthyliving/the-dangers-of-sitting.

[7] the website for Mayo Clinic Health System, "The Importance of Moving"; https://www.mayoclinichealthsystem.org/hometown-health/featured-topic/the-importance-of-movement; by Andrew Jagim, Ph.D., posted June 8, 2020.

[8] Lipman and Greeven, *How to Be Well*, 121.

[9] the website for Mayo Clinic Health System, The Importance of Movement"; https://www.mayoclinichealthsystem.org/hometown-health/featured-topic/the-importance-of-movement; by Andrew Jagim, Ph.D., posted June 8, 2020.

[10] Ornish and Ornish, *UnDo It!*, 103.

[11] Sherzai and Sherzai, *The Alzheimer's Solution*, 147.

[12] Ornish and Ornish, *UnDo It!*, 104.

[13] the website for CDC Centers for Disease Control and Prevention; Division of Nutrition, Physical Activity and Obesity, National Center for Chronic Disease Prevention and Health Promotion."How Much Physical Activity Do Older Adults Need"; https://www.cdc.gov/physicalactivity/basics/older adults/index.htm ; Last Reviewed April 13, 2023.

[14] the website for CDC Centers for Disease Control and Prevention; Division of Nutrition, Physical Activity and Obesity, National Center for Chronic Disease Prevention and Health Promotion."How Much Physical Activity Do Older Adults Need"; https://www.cdc.gov/physicalactivity/basics/older adults/index.htm ; Last Reviewed April 13, 2023.

[15] the website for health.gov, U.S. Department of Health and Human Services; "Physical Activity Guidelines for Americans, 2nd Ed. https://health.gov/sites/

default/files/2019-09/Physical_Activity_Guidelines_2nd_edition.pdf#page=56.

[16] the website for CDC Centers for Disease Control and Prevention; Division of Nutrition, Physical Activity and Obesity, National Center for Chronic Disease Prevention and Health Promotion; "How Much Physical ACTIVITY Do Older Adults Need? https://www.cdc.gov/physicalactivity/basics/olderadults/index.htm.

[17] the website for health.gov, U.S. Department of Health and Human Services; "Physical Activity Guidelines for Americans, 2nd Ed; Spotlight on Aerobic Activities: A Tried and Try Favorite and Two Increasingly Popular Options. Talk Test" https://health.gov/sites/default/files/2019-09/Physical_Activity_Guidelines_2nd_edition.pdf#page=60.

[18] Ornish and Ornish, *UnDo It!*, 104-105.

[19] Janis Tremaine, email message to author (Omlie), June 29, 2022.

[20] Saray Stancic MD, *What's Missing from Medicine. Six Lifestyle Changes to Overcome Chronic Illness* (San Antonio: Hicrophant Publishing, 2021), xxv-xxxii.

[21] Gigi Carter, email message to author (Omlie), July 29, 2022.

[22] the website for CDC Centers for Disease Control and Prevention; Division of Nutrition, Physical Activity and Obesity, National Center for Chronic Disease Prevention and Health Promotion; "How Much Physical Activity Do Adults Need? Some Activity is Better Than None," https://www.cdc.gov/physicalactivity/basics/adults/index.htm.

Chapter 8

[1] Cheryl Richardson, *The Art of Extreme Self-Care. 12 Practical and Inspiring Ways to Love Yourself More* (Carlsbad: Hay House, Inc., 2019), 67.

[2] Richardson, *The Art of Extreme Self-Care*, 68.

[3] the website for Psychology Today. Addiction; "Six Steps to Stop and Addiction to Sugar and Junk Food" https://www.psychologytoday.com/us/blog/advancing-psychiatry/201906/six-steps-stop-addiction-sugar-and-junk-food; by Christopher M. Palmer, MD, Reviewed by Ekua Hagan, Posted June 11, 2019.

[4] Neal Barnard, MD, *Your Body in Balance. The New Science of Food, Hormones, and Health* (New York; Grand Central Publishing, 2020), 217-226.

[5] Barnard, *Your Body in Balance*, 229-230.

[6] Barnard, *Your Body in Balance*, 234-235.

[7] Deepak Chopra MD and Kimberly Snyder CN, *Radical Beauty, How to Transform Yourself from Inside Out (*New York: Harmony Books, 2016), 114.

[8] AllSides has a great media bias chart that classifies news sources on a spectrum from left to right. The website for "AllSides. Don't Be Fooled by Media Bias and Misinformation" "AllSides Media Bias Chart"; https://www.allsides.com/media-bias/media-bias-chart.

Chapter 9

[1] Sherrie Campbell, Ph.D., "The 10 Understated Qualities of Beauty," as published in *Arizona Health & Living,* Aug. 2017, p.32 & 33. Reprinted with permission from Sherrie Campbell, Ph.D. and Lisa Padilla, publisher Arizona Health & Living.

Acknowledgments

I want to acknowledge several people who have inspired me to write this book.

First and foremost, I want to thank Dr. T. Colin Campbell for his research and perseverance in the whole food, plant-based concept. Without it, I would be dead right now or suffering from many of the chronic diseases that are plaguing us today. I know his journey has been challenging and unpopular. So, thank you, Dr. Campbell!

Second, I want to thank Rip Esselstyn. He is another pioneer who paved the way for me to learn and integrate a whole-food, plant-based diet into my life and make the vast changes that needed to be made. From his initial book to his enlightening podcast, which I continue to listen to today, thank you, Rip!

—*Debbye Omlie*

Thank you, Brandi, for your inspiration and encouragement. My contribution to this book would not have happened without you. Because of you, I strive to be a better person, a better man, a better husband, and a better father. I am so excited about the life we have created together!

And thanks to Debbye for thinking of me to contribute to your book. Your hard work laid the foundation for the book and made it easy for me to seamlessly blend my thoughts into a cohesive narrative. I am so grateful for the opportunity you gave me!

— *Blake Anderson*

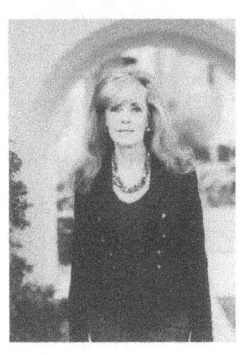

About Debbye

Debbye Omlie started learning about healthy living principles in her early thirties. She started a worksite wellness program for a Honeywell division, heralded by the American Heart Association as a model in New Mexico. With a passion for health, she has worked in communications, marketing, public relations, and events for numerous healthcare organizations promoting healthy living principles for over fifteen years.

But when her family started dying from preventable lifestyle-related diseases, Omlie knew she had to find a better way to live. This book is the result of her research into scientific, evidence-based information. This is a healthy aging beginner's manual with information about where one can start and how to create a customized plan for yourself.

Omlie earned a Master of Mass Communication degree from Arizona State University, Walter Cronkite School of Journalism and Mass Communication and a Bachelor of Business Administration degree from the University of Mary Hardin-Baylor.

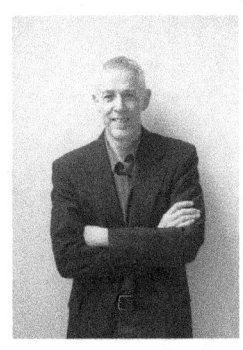

About Blake

Born and raised in the Pacific Northwest, Blake Anderson earned his B.S. in Mathematics from the University of Washington and turned that into a successful thirty-year career in the tech industry, over twenty of which were spent at Microsoft, working in various teams from Office to Bing to Xbox.

Blake's health journey started when he discovered himself overweight and out of shape. He was able to turn his health around through small, but meaningful, changes that led to the results he wanted to see. The lifestyle changes stuck and so did the results! While in the midst of his health transformation, he was beset by personal tragedy. After struggling for many years, he re-imagined a better future for himself and, through creativity and persistence, was able to build a new life out of the ashes his old life had become.

Driven by his own personal success and fueled by a passion to help others, Blake started his own Life and Wellness Coaching business called Honu Perspective. He has a Wellness Coaching certification from the Mayo Clinic and Breakthrough Coaching and Neuro-Transformational Coaching certifications from Elite Coaching University. He enjoys helping clients work through their fears, limiting beliefs, and other resistance to change, empowering them to accomplish their goals and achieve a more balanced life and greater sense of well-being.

Blake currently lives in Kirkland, Washington, with his beautiful wife, Brandi, and their precious little newborn, Braelyn.

www.ingramcontent.com/pod-product-compliance
Lightning Source LLC
LaVergne TN
LVHW011842060526
838200LV00054B/4139